The
TOXICOLOGY HANDBOOK
for CLINICIANS

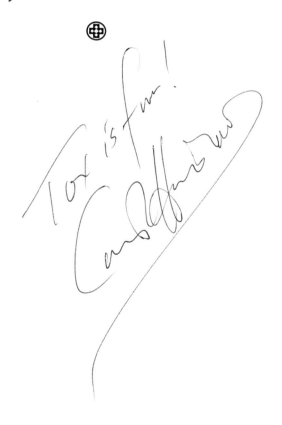

Tox is fun!

The TOXICOLOGY HANDBOOK for CLINICIANS

CARSON R. HARRIS, MD
Senior Staff Emergency Physician
Director, Clinical Toxicology Consulting Service
Emergency Medicine Department
Regions Hospital
St. Paul, Minnesota
Associate Professor
Department of Emergency Medicine
University of Minnesota Medical School
Assistant Clinical Professor, College of Pharmacy
University of Minnesota
Consultant for the Hennepin Regional Poison Center
Minneapolis, Minnesota

MOSBY
ELSEVIER

MOSBY
ELSEVIER

1600 John F. Kennedy Blvd.
Suite 1800
Philadelphia, PA 19103-2899

THE TOXICOLOGY HANDBOOK FOR CLINICIANS

Library of Congress Cataloging-in-Publication Data
1-56053-711-6
Acquisitions Editor: Todd Hummel
Project Manager: Mary Stermel
Marketing Manager: Matt Latuchie

Printed in the United States of America.

Last digit is the print number: 9   8   7   6   5   4   3   2   1

Acknowledgments

I would like to acknowledge the hard work and dedication of the authors who help bring this project to fruition. I am truly grateful for their efforts in the midst of their busy schedules. I would also like to thank my wife, Maren, and children, Taylor, Whitney and Drew for their encouragement, support and understanding.

Contributors

Beth Baker, MD, MPH
Occupational and Environmental Medicine
Regions Hospital
St. Paul, Minnesota

Marny Benjamin, MD
Staff Physician, Emergency Medicine
Methodist Hospital
St. Louis Park, Minnesota

Scott Cameron, MD
Staff Physician, Emergency Medicine
Whangarei, New Zealand

David Cheesebrow, RN, CCN
Staff Registered Nurse, Emergency Medicine
Emergency Medicine Department
Regions Hospital
St. Paul, Minnesota

Chanah DeLisle, MD
Staff Attending Physician
Suburban Emergency Associates
St. Francis Region Medical Center
Shakopee, Minnesota

Kristin Engebretsen, PharmD
Clinical Toxicologist, Clinical Toxicology Service
Emergency Medicine Department
Regions Hospital
St. Paul, Minnesota

Bradley Gordon, MD
Emergency Physician
Emergency Medicine Department
Regions Hospital
St. Paul, Minnesota

Carson R. Harris, MD
Director, Clinical Toxicology Service
Emergency Medicine Department
Regions Hospital
St. Paul, Minnesota

Bradley Hernandez, MD
Senior Staff Physician
Emergency Medicine Department
Regions Hospital
St. Paul, Minnesota

Joel S. Holger, MD
Senior Staff Physician
Emergency Medicine Department
Regions Hospital
St. Paul, Minnesota

Peter Kumasaka, MD
Senior Staff Physician
Emergency Medicine Department
Regions Hospital
St. Paul, Minnesota

Richard P. Lamon, MD
Senior Staff Physician
Emergency Medicine Department
Regions Hospital
St. Paul, Minnesota

Michael McGrail, MD, MPH
Occupational and Environmental Medicine
Regions Hospital
St. Paul, Minnesota

Kathleen A. Neacy, MD
Senior Staff Physician
Emergency Medicine Department
Regions Hospital
St. Paul, Minnesota

Christopher S. Russi, MD
Associate Director, Emergency Medicine
Residency Program, Clinical Assistant
Professor, Department of Emergency Medicine
University of Iowa

Steven C. Wandersee, PA-C
Lead Physician Assistant, Emergency Medicine
Emergency Medicine Department
Regions Hospital
St. Paul, Minnesota

James P. Winter, MD, RPh
Staff Attending, Emergency Medicine
Emergency Associates and Consulting
Coeur d'Alene, Idaho

Stephanie Witt, MD
Emergency Medicine Faculty
MetroHealth Medical Center
Cleveland, Ohio

James Wood, MD
Staff Attending, Emergency Medicine
Emergency Medicine Department
Kaiser Permanente
Portland, Oregon

Preface

Alle Ding' sind Gift und nichts ohn' Gift; allein die Dosis macht, das ein Ding kein Gift ist. ["All things are poison and nothing (is) without poison; only the dose makes that a thing is no poison."] – Paracelsus, the Father of Toxicology

Toxicology is defined as the study of the nature, effects, and detection of poisons and the treatment of poisoning. Either in the clinic setting, emergency department, or on hospital wards, clinicians encounter patients with toxic effects of drugs and chemicals, or the interactions of multiple drugs leading to toxic effects. In many cases the effects are due to overdose, either intentional or accidental. To deal with these cases we have prepared a handbook to outline the pertinent information on the common and interesting drugs and chemicals encountered. Each chapter contains key pearls and pitfalls related to the drug or toxin. This section of the chapter is to increase your knowledge and obviate classic mistakes in management. To assist in decision-making we have included some of the admission criteria, however, clinical judgment should prevail and any error in judgment should be made in the patient's favor.

In addition, this handbook contain appendices to help you remember some of the important aspects of toxicology, understand the function of your toxicology laboratory, and an extensive list of street names and terms for drugs of abuse, which are ever-present and seems to touch all clinical practices.

It is our intent to provide an easy-to-read, useful handbook for quick information on toxicology patients. This is not intended to be a major reference manual, as there are several suggested readings for each chapter if you want to gain a deeper understanding of the topic and when you have time. It is my hope that this handbook will be useful to the medical student, hospital and emergency department residents, and hospital and clinic attendings.

Remember, Tox is Fun!

Carson R. Harris, MD

Table of Contents

Section I

Common Ingestions and Exposures You Might See

Section II

Special Tox Conditions

Section III

Toxicology Mnemonics and Useful Pearls

Common

INGESTIONS AND

Exposures YOU MIGHT SEE

Management Strategies in Overdoses: The ABCs of Toxicology

The list of drugs and toxins that a patient can ingest in an overdose are numerous. Not all drugs and toxins have antidotes to reverse the toxic effects, but a few general principles might get you through the initial phase of management. In emergency medicine and critical patients we typically start resuscitation with ABCs, Airway, Breathing and Circulation. However in an overdose scenario, the ABCs are somewhat different and provides more of a focus on the ingestion.

Management Strategies. The ABCDEs of toxicology are applied after the Emergency Medicine Safety Net (Oxygen, IV access, ECG Monitor) is in place.

The A is *Antidote*. If you know that there is an antidote, give it early.

Common Antidote	Overdose/Toxin
Oxygen	Carbon monoxide, cyanide, hydrogen sulfide
Naloxone	Narcotics/opiates
Atropine, pralidoxime	Organophosphates
NAC	Acetaminophen, carbon tetrachloride
Calcium	Hydrofluoric acid, fluorides, oxalates
DMSA	Lead (FDA approval), arsenic, mercury
Sodium bicarbonate	TCA (tricyclic antidepressants)
Fab fragments	Digoxin (DigiFab/Digibind), cardiac glycoside plants (foxglove, oleander)
Ethanol, fomepizole	Ethylene glycol, methanol
Physostigmine	Anticholinergic (central effects)
Pyridoxine	INH

B is, apply the *Basics*

Insure the usual Airway, Breathing, and Circulation is accomplished.

C is *Charcoal*.

Usually, 50-100 g for adults and 1 g/kg in pediatrics.

The recommendation for treating toxic ingestions with single-dose activated charcoal is that it is more beneficial if given **within 60 min of a potentially toxic ingestion.** Remember, activated charcoal does not ADsorb metals (iron, lithium, potassium) or alcohols very well. Also, it should not be given in caustic and hydrocarbon ingestions.

Multiple doses of AC (MDAC) may be given in certain ODs (aspirin, enteric coated or sustained released preparations, TCAs, Phenobarbital or theophylline). This is accomplished by a full dose followed by $\frac{1}{2}$ doses every 2-4 hr. In most cases, three to four doses are given. However, drugs receiving the best support in the literature for effective MDAC treatment are phenobarbital, theophylline, quinine, dapsone, and carbamazepine.

D is *Decontamination* procedures such as gastric lavage, or irrigation.

For gastric lavage, this procedure has not been shown to change the course or outcome of ingestions if done more than 60 min post ingestion. It is recommended to do gastric lavage if the patient presents within 60 min of a potentially lethal ingestion of a substance. Gastric lavage is not a benign procedure and may increase morbidity. Esophageal injuries and aspiration are some of our biggest worries with this procedure. Technique is very important in maximizing effectiveness and yield. Endotracheal intubation may be necessary in obtunded patients. Placing the patient on his or her left side and head down 20–30 degrees may help prevent aspiration and improve the yield of the procedure.

Ipecac syrup and cathartics have not been shown to be of benefit in overdoses. If ipecac is recommended, it is usually done so by the Poison Center and given in the home (very early after the ingestion).

E is *Enhanced elimination.*

This includes hemodialysis, hemoperfusion, whole bowel lavage, pH manipulation (urine or blood, or both), and other adjunct therapeutic modalities that may be useful in toxic situations.

There are relatively few overdoses that are effectively managed by hemodialysis, but traditionally the following drugs have been referred for hemodialysis treatment: Salicylates, Theophylline, Methanol, Meprobamate, Metoprolol, Barbiturates (esp. long-acting), Lithium, Ethylene Glycol (antifreeze), Valproate.

Generally, following the ABCDEs of toxicology and consultation your regional poison center (1-800-222-1222) or local toxicologist are the best strategies in managing the overdose patient.

When discussing your toxicology case with the toxicologist or Poison Center, it is helpful to remember that the Tox history really "MATtERS"

> M is *Medications* or *Materials* ingested or exposed to
> A is *Amount* ingested or the concentration of the material if known
> Tt is *Time taken* or approximate time of exposure
> E is *Emesis* with or without pill fragments or chemical residue
> R is for *Reason* for the ingestion or exposure. Accidental or unintentional ingestions tend to be less worrisome depending on the type of product. International, homicidal, or assaults with poisons or drugs are more worrisome.
> S is *Signs* and *symptoms* you have noticed or the patient complains of during your evaluation.

This information along with your laboratory test results, ECG, and radiographs (if obtained) will help the toxicologist during the phone conversation.

Chapter 1

Salicylates (Aspirin)

Richard P. Lamon

▮ Overview

Aspirin, the first nonsteroidal anti-inflammatory drug (NSAID), was first used in 1899 and is still a life-threatening overdose. It is used and prescribed as an anti-inflammatory, antipyretic, and analgesic drug. In addition, millions of people use aspirin as a platelet-aggregation inhibitor.

Salicylates are ubiquitous in their distribution. They are found individually or in combination as tablets, capsules, powders, effervescent tablets, liquids, liniments, creams, and lotions.

They are also found in sunscreens, topical antiarthritics, herbal Chinese medicines, nonaspirin salicylates, plants (e.g., acacia flower oil, aspens, birches, camellias [leaves], hyacinths, marigolds, milkwort, poplars, spirea, teaberries, tulips, and violets), and foods (e.g., almonds, apples, apricots, blackberries, cherries, grapes, nectarines, oranges, peaches, plums, and raspberries).

Salicylates may be enteric-coated or sustained-release preparations.

The Done nomogram, previously used to determine toxicity, is no longer clinically useful. Use of the nomogram may overestimate or underestimate acute salicylate poisoning and is not helpful with chronic toxicity or with extended release products.

Decisions on management of acute salicylate overdose should be based on clinical presentation and good judgment as well as the serum salicylate concentration in relation to the time of ingestion.

Toxicity

Toxicity can occur from ingestion or dermal exposure. In addition, toxic substances can be absorbed rectally.

Substances

- Methylsalicylate (oil of wintergreen) can contain 98% of methylsalicylate and 1 mL is equivalent to 1.4 g of acetylsalicylic acid (ASA) in salicylate potency.
- Bismuth subsalicylate is found in antidiarrheals (8.77 mg salicylic acid/mL).
- Topical salicylates include homomenthyl salicylates (46% salicylic acid), which are found in sunscreens.

Clinical Presentation

Acute Ingestions

- **Less than 150 mg/kg**: Asymptomatic to mild toxicity
- **150–300 mg/kg**: Mild to moderate toxicity
  - Signs and symptoms may include fever, tachypnea, tinnitus, respiratory alkalosis, metabolic acidosis, lethargy, mild dehydration, nausea, and vomiting.
- **300–500 mg/kg**: Severe toxicity
  - Signs and symptoms may include encephalopathy, coma, hypotension, pulmonary edema, seizures, acidemia, coagulopathy, cerebral edema, and dysrhythmias.
  - Central nervous system (CNS) signs and symptoms dominate clinically, with signs of stimulation followed by CNS depression (i.e., confusion, delirium, and psychosis leading to stupor, convulsions, and coma).
  - Serious signs of severe toxicity include cardiac dysrhythmias, noncardiogenic pulmonary edema, acute renal failure, hemorrhage, increased or decreased blood sugar, ketonemia, and ketonuria.
- **Greater than 500 mg/kg**: Potentially lethal

Chronic Ingestions

- Most commonly seen in older adults and infants (e.g., over-treatment of fever)*
- Polypharmacy ingestions in which the patient may be taking more than one salicylate-containing medication or drug interaction (Chinese medications, acetazolamide, alcohol)
- Suspect with unexplained CNS dysfunction with mixed acid–base disturbance, anion gap acidosis (remember "MUDPILES")
- Change in mentation is the usual presenting complaint (i.e., confusion, disorientation, lethargy, or hallucinations).
- Respiratory alkalosis with anion gap metabolic acidosis and a normal or increased pH is the most frequent acid–base abnormality.
- Noncardiac pulmonary edema is common in chronic overdose.
- Vital signs
  - Increased respirations, heart rate, and temperature are common in mild to moderate toxicity.
  - Decreased blood pressure suggests severe toxicity.
- HEENT
  - Tinnitus, decreased hearing, and electrocochleographic changes may occur with high therapeutic levels and overdoses.
- Cardiovascular
  - Tachycardia with mild to moderate toxicity
  - Hypotension and dysrhythmias with severe toxicity
- Respiratory
  - Tachypnea and hypercapnea are common.
  - Noncardiogenic pulmonary edema may be seen in cases of severe toxicity.
- Neurologic
  - Lethargy, agitation, and confusion are early signs of severe toxicity.
  - Coma, seizures, and cerebral edema are late signs of severe toxicity.
- Gastrointestinal (GI)
  - Nausea and vomiting are common.
  - GI bleeding, perforation, and pancreatitis are rare in acute overdose.

---

*Aspirin is rarely recommended for pediatric fever because of an association with Reye's syndrome.

- GI bleeding and perforation are more common in **chronic overdose.**
- Hepatic
  - Chronic toxicity and chronic therapeutic use can cause elevated transaminases.
  - Remember, salicylates are associated with Reye's syndrome.
- Genitourinary
  - Renal insufficiency is uncommon but more frequently occurs secondary to decreased blood pressure or rhabdomyolysis.
- Acid base
  - Produces anion gap acidosis (normal gap is 15 or less); Anion gap = $Na - (Cl + HCO_3)$.
  - **Respiratory alkalosis** occurs early and may be the only sign of mild salicylism.
  - Compensatory metabolic acidosis develops in most adults with moderate intoxication.
  - **Metabolic acidosis** with acidemia and compensatory respiratory alkalosis in severe overdoses
    - Increased rate of complications and death
    - K^+ and HCO_3 depletion occur with shift in H^+ to the extracellular space.
    - Results in an acidic blood pH and acidic urine pH
    - Acidemia increases the nonionized fraction of salicylates and salicylate distribution to tissues (increased CNS and pulmonary toxicity and higher mortality rate).
  - **Infants:** Respiratory alkalosis may be short lived or not occur at all. Metabolic acidosis with acidemia predominates.
- Gynecologic
  - Chronic maternal use is associated with increased incidence of stillbirth, antepartum and postpartum bleeding, prolonged pregnancy, and labor with low-birth-weight infant.
  - Pregnancy Category D
- Fluid and electrolytes
  - Dehydration secondary to fever, diaphoresis, hyperpnea, vomiting, and decreased PO intake (particularly in chronic toxicity)
  - Decreased K^+ is common and may worsen with attempts at alkaline diuresis.
- Hematologic
  - PT prolongation is fairly common in chronic intoxication.
  - DIC and thrombocytopenia are rare.

▋ Laboratory Evaluation

Obtain salicylate level.

- Initial level is useful in determining diagnosis.
- Serum salicylate levels peak more rapidly after methylsalicylate (oil of wintergreen) ingestions, more slowly with large amounts that form concretions and more slowly yet with enteric-coated and sustained-release preparations.
- Remember the following:
  - Nontoxic levels (<30 mg/dL) <6 hr postingestion do not rule out impending toxicity.
  - Massive overdoses may be toxic before 6-hr level for nomogram (i.e., massive salicylate ingestion or methylsalicylate).
  - Chronic ingestions may have therapeutic level on nomogram. Serum level does not correlate with blood gas analysis or patient's mentation. Therefore in cases of chronic toxicity, accurate lab assessment of the severity of toxicity is impossible.
- Ferric chloride test (qualitative test)
  - Helpful in determining whether salicylates are present, but not helpful in management
  - Place a few drops of 10% $FeCl_2$ in 1 mL of urine. It will turn purple in the presence of even small quantities of salicylate.
  - False-positive result with acetoacetic acid and phenylpyruvic acid
  - Ferric chloride test is preferred to Ames Phenistix because the color change is easier to detect.
- Ames Phenistix turns brown with salicylate or phenothiazine.

The following tests are used to monitor the patient:

- Monitor salicylate level, glucose, and electrolytes every 2 hr until salicylate level is consistently falling and acid–base abnormalities are improving.
- Arterial blood gases (ABGs): Perform in symptomatic patients and follow until acid–base abnormalities improve. ABGs determine the type and severity (degree) of acid–base imbalance.
- Complete blood count (CBC), renal function tests, liver function tests (LFTs), International Normalized Ratio (INR), prothrombin time (PT), and partial thromboplastin time (PTT) in patients with clinical evidence of toxicity
- Chest radiograph if hypoxic or signs or symptoms of pulmonary edema

- Abdominal radiograph if concern about bezoars or
  concretions (concretions of enteric-coated bismuth
  subsalicylate may be radiopaque on plain films); may also
  use contrast if bezoars or concretions are concerns

Treatment

Dermal Exposure

Cleanse skin with soap and water.

Oral-Parenteral Exposure

- Decontamination
  - Ipecac: Not indicated in hospital management of
    overdose
  - Gastric lavage may be indicated if patient presents less
    than 1 hr after potentially life-threatening ingestion
    of substances known to form bezoars or concretions.
    Protect airway. Should not be considered routine in all
    poisoned patients.
- Activated charcoal
  - 25–100 g in adults (0.5–1.0 g/kg)
  - 25–50 g in 1- to 12-year-old children
  - 1 g/kg in infants younger than 12 months
- Whole bowel irrigation: Helpful with sustained-release
  preparations and enteric-coated forms
  - Correct dehydration and electrolyte abnormalities.
  - Normal saline at rate of 10–20 mL/kg/hr over 1–2 hr
    until good urine flow is obtained (1–2 mL/kg/hr)
  - Once good urine flow is obtained, potassium should be
    added to IV fluids (20–40 mEq/L).
- Monitor and correct hypoglycemia.
  - Patient may exhibit CNS glucopenia even in the pres-
    ence of a normal peripheral glucose.
  - Any change in mental status should prompt a consider-
    ation of giving glucose (i.e., D50).
  - Alkalinize the serum and urine in patients with clinical
    or laboratory evidence of toxicity (salicylate levels greater
    than 50–60 mEq/dL on a 6-hr level).
- Administer bolus of 1–2 mEq/kg NaHCO$_3$ followed by a
  continuous infusion of the following: 2–3 amps of NaHCO$_3$
  in a liter of D5W infused at 1.5× to 2× maintenance fluid
  requirements to achieve a urine pH greater than 7.5. May
  need additional KCl to obtain alkaline urine.

- Hemodialysis indications
  - Blood salicylate level greater than 100 mg/dL or salicylate level <100 mg/dL plus:
  - Refractory acidosis
  - Persistent CNS symptoms (e.g., encephalopathy, coma, seizures, altered mental status, or cerebral edema), especially in chronic ingestions
  - Progressive clinical deterioration despite appropriate therapy or inability to achieve alkalinization of urine
  - Pulmonary edema or acute respiratory distress syndrome (ARDS)
  - Renal failure
  - **Do not rely on blood levels alone to determine the need for dialysis.**

Special Considerations

Pregnancy and Lactation

- Pregnancy Category D
  - Pregnancy Category D means: "There is positive evidence of human fetal risk based on adverse reaction data from investigational or marketing experience or studies in humans, but potential benefits may warrant use of the drug in pregnant women despite potential risks." The Physicians Desk Reference gives it a category X, meaning: "Studies in animals or humans have demonstrated fetal abnormalities and/or there is positive evidence of human fetal risk based on adverse reaction data from investigational or marketing experience, and the risks involved in use of the drug in pregnant women clearly outweigh potential benefits."
- Secreted in breast milk
- The American Academy of Pediatrics recommends that breastfeeding mothers use aspirin cautiously during lactation because of its potential adverse affects to the nursing infant.

Admission Criteria

- All patients with major signs or symptoms: acidosis, dehydration, mental status changes, seizures, or pulmonary edema, regardless of the salicylate level (see notes concerning chronic salicylate toxicity)

- All suspected chronic poisonings, infants and children under the age of 2 years, older adults, chronic overdoses, enteric-coated overdoses, and sustained-release overdoses
- Suicide ingestions on medicine ward or psychiatry unit depending on clinical clearance

Pearls and Pitfalls

- Failure to consider the diagnosis in cases of chronic salicylate toxicity is a common pitfall.
- More than 50% of cases are misdiagnosed at the time of admission.
- Consider salicylate toxicity in any older adult with unexpected delirium or fever.
- Consider dialysis early in patients who are ill and in those without early improvement to supportive care (e.g., severe acidosis, hypokalemia).
- Give glucose in altered mental states even if the patient is euglycemic.

References and Suggested Readings

1. Anderson RJ, Potts DE, Gabow PA, et al: Unrecognized adult salicylate intoxication, *Ann Intern Med* 85:745-748, 1976.
2. Bailey RB, Jones SR: Chronic salicylate intoxication: a common cause of morbidity in the elderly, *J Am Geriatr Soc* 37:556-561, 1989.
3. Done AK: Aspirin overdose: incidence, diagnosis, and management, *Pediatrics* 62(suppl):890-897, 1978.
4. Azer M, Bailey H: www.emedicine.com/MED/topic2057.htm. emedicine from WebMD.
5. Gittelman DK: Chronic salicylate intoxication, *South Med J* 86:683-385, 1993.
6. Goldfrank LR, Weisman RS, Flomenbaum NE, et al, eds: *Goldfrank's toxicologic emergencies,* ed 5, Norwalk, CT, 1994, Appleton & Lange.
7. Salicylates, Micromedex® Healthcare Series, Poisindex®, Vol 128, expired June 2006.
8. Dugandzic RM, Tierney MG, Dickinson GE, et al: Evaluation of the validity of the Done nomogram in the management of acute salicylate intoxication. *Ann Emerg Med* 18(11):1186-1190, 1989.

Chapter 2

Acetaminophen

Richard P. Lamon

Overview

Acetaminophen is the most widely used analgesic in the world. It is contained in more than 100 different products and is available as liquids, tablets, chewables, suspensions, suppositories, and in combination with other medications such as narcotics, caffeine, and antihistamines. It is also available as extended-release preparations. Acetaminophen is the most common drug associated with intentional and accidental poisoning.

Substances

Also known as APAP, paracetamol, paracetamolum, 4-hydroxyacetanilide, and N-acetyl-p-aminophenol.

Toxicity

- Rapidly absorbed from the stomach and intestines into the bloodstream
- Metabolized in the liver by conjugation to nontoxic agents, which are eliminated in urine
- In an acute overdose or when maximal daily dose is exceeded for more than 3 days, the normal pathways of metabolism become saturated, and excess acetaminophen is metabolized in the liver by the P450 system to become

a toxic metabolite, *N*-acetyl-p-benzoquinone-imine (NAPQI). NAPQI, which has a short half-life, is rapidly conjugated with glutathione, a sulfhydryl donor, and removed from the system. Under conditions of excessive NAPQI formation or reduced glutathione stores, NAPQI is free to covalently bind to vital proteins and the lipid layer of hepatocytes, resulting in hepatocellular death and subsequent centrilobular liver necrosis.

- Maximal daily dose is 4 g in adults and 90 mg/kg in children.
- Toxic dose in a single acute ingestion is 150 mg/kg or 7.5 g in adults.
- Toxic dose is believed to be lower in people with alcoholism, acquired immunodeficiency syndrome (AIDS), malnutrition, and anorexia nervosa because of decreased glutathione stores and inadequate detoxifying of NAPQI. However, this association is controversial.
- Patients with enhanced ability to make NAPQI because of induction of the P450 system may be at increased risk of morbidity, including people who take rifampin, phenobarbital, isoniazid, phenytoin, or carbamazepine or those who chronically abuse alcohol.
- Children who are less than 12 years old appear to fare better than adults, possibly because of their increased capacity to conjugate acetaminophen, enhanced detoxification of NAPQI, or increased glutathione stores. However, this has not been proven by controlled studies, and children should be treated the same as adults.

▮ Clinical Presentation

See Table 2-1.
The four phases of acetaminophen poisoning are as follows:
- Phase 1 (0–24 hr [Day 1]): asymptomatic, anorexia, nausea and vomiting, diaphoresis, malaise
- Phase 2 (18–72 hr [Days 2–3]): decrease in the symptoms of Phase 1, RUQ pain and increased liver enzymes (i.e., alanine transaminase [ALT] and aspartate aminotransferase [AST])
- Phase 3 (72–96 hr [Days 3–4]): centrilobular hepatic necrosis with accompanying abdominal pain, jaundice, coagulopathy, hepatic encephalopathy, recurrence of nausea and vomiting, renal failure, and fatality
- Phase 4 (4 days to 3 weeks): complete resolution of symptoms or organ failure

Table 2-1 CLINICAL PRESENTATION AND FINDINGS

System	Clinical Findings
Hepatic	Main toxicity, severe, life-threatening. Most common cause of hepatic failure that requires transplant. Evidence of hepatotoxicity usually observed 24–48 hr postingestion, elevation of transaminases, central lobular necrosis, hyperbilirubinemia, hepatic failure but can occur as early as 16–18 hr postingestion
Cardiovascular	Myocardial injury (rarely)
Respiratory	Noncardiogenic pulmonary edema in severe poisoning
Neurologic	Coma and metabolic acidosis in severe poisoning
Gastrointestinal	Nausea and vomiting early or late, right upper quadrant abdominal pain with liver injury, increased amylase, and gastrointestinal hemorrhage with hepatotoxicity
Genitourinary	Transient renal damage, acute tubular necrosis, flank pain, hematuria, proteinuria, and anti-diuretic hormone effect (usually in severe toxicity)
Acid base	Increase lactate levels; metabolic acidosis in patients that develop hepatic failure
Fluid or electrolytes	Decreased phosphate level (possibly)
Endocrine	Hypoglycemia with hepatotoxicity
Reproductive	Category B. Crosses placental barrier. Fetal blood level will probably be as high or higher than maternal. No evidence that normal doses of acetaminophen represent a risk to the fetus or nursing infant
Hematologic	Prolonged prothrombin time, thrombocytopenia, bleeding; acetaminophen does not cause methemoglobinemia-like phenacetin

Laboratory Evaluation

- Obtaining a plasma acetaminophen level is important for diagnosis and treatment even in the absence of symptoms.
- Check the acetaminophen level in any intentional overdose because the history is often unreliable and manifestations of toxicity may not become evident until after treatment would have been initiated.
- Obtain the 4-hr postingestion acetaminophen level; earlier levels cannot predict the potential of hepatotoxicity or need for antidotal therapy with *N*-acetylcysteine (NAC).
- Plot the level on the Rumack-Matthew nomogram* as a guide to NAC treatment.

The nomogram is not helpful before 4 hr or after 24 hr or in cases of multiple acetaminophen ingestions, polydrug ingestions (including acetaminophen) that may affect the absorption of acetaminophen, extended-release acetaminophen preparations, or chronic ingestions.

- Remember, the history of time of ingestion, quantity and formulation of acetaminophen ingested, and coingestants is important but often unreliable.
- Other laboratory tests are ordered as indicated (see the next section) and as needed for evaluation of coingestants at the time of presentation.
- If the acetaminophen level is in the toxic range, obtain serum glutamic-oxaloacetic transaminase (SGOT [ALT]), serum glutamate pyruvate transaminase (SGPT [ALT]), total bilirubin, protime, blood urea nitrogen (BUN), and creatinine on admittance, repeat the tests daily for 3 days or until these levels begin a consistent downward trend.
- If the liver function tests are increased, check electrolytes, glucose, blood urea nitrogen (BUN), creatinine, urinalysis, hemoglobin (Hgb), hematocrit (HCT), amylase, and EKG as clinically indicated.
- Human chorionic gonadotropin (HCG) should be checked in all women of childbearing age, type and cross if active bleeding and arterial blood gas (ABG) if evidence of mental status changes or level >600 µg/mL.
- Consider computerized tomography (CT) scan of head if mental status changes.

▐ Treatment

- Antidotal therapy is most effective when initiated within 8 hr postingestion.

Acute Ingestions

- Lavage is rarely indicated in acetaminophen ingestions unless there is a concomitant life-threatening co-ingestion and the patient presents within 60 min (or later if the life threatening co-ingestion forms concretions).
- Emesis is **not recommended** in emergency departments; may delay administration of NAC, charcoal, or both. Minimally efficient and not very effective when given in the ED.
  - Emesis may be used in home situations to prevent absorption.

- Give **activated charcoal** when patient presents within 1–2 hr postingestion.
  - Adults: 1 g/kg PO or 10 times the amount of ingested drug
  - Children: as in adults
- NAC is the drug of choice for prevention and treatment of acetaminophen-induced hepatotoxicity. It is given PO or IV for patients who cannot tolerate PO secondary to vomiting.
  - Most effective when given within 8 hr of ingestion. However, NAC should be considered whenever hepato-toxicity secondary to acetaminophen is evident, regardless of the time postingestion.
  - NAC is supplied as a 20% solution. For PO, dilute to 5% solution in juice or a cola soft drink.

NAC Administration

Oral Administration: Adults
- **Loading dose** of 140 mg/kg orally as 5% solution in soft drink or juice. May use NG tube to administer.
- **Maintenance dose** of 70 mg/kg orally as 5% solution every 4 hr for a total of 17 doses over 72 hr
- Abbreviated oral NAC dosing of 24–48 hours has also been used. Discuss this with your toxicologist or Poison Center.
- Consider giving antiemetic prior to the NAC.

Oral Administration: Children
- Administer as in adults.
- Consider giving antiemetic prior to the NAC.

IV Administration: Adults

On January 23, 2004 Cumberland Pharmaceuticals, Inc. received FDA approval for Acetadote, the first IV formulation of acetylcysteine for use in the Emergency Room setting to prevent or lessen potential liver damage resulting from overdose of acetaminophen, the leading cause of drug toxicity in the United States. Acetadote is the first injectable treatment FDA approved for treatment of acetaminophen overdose available in the United States. Previously Mucomyst (Apothecon, Inc.) was used without FDA approval.

ACETADOTE: IV ADMINISTRATION: ADULTS (≥40 kg)
  Three-Bag Method
- Estimate time of acetaminophen ingestion

- Less than 24 hr since overdose
- Draw serum for acetaminophen level at 4 hr post-ingestion or as soon as possible thereafter, PLOT LEVEL ON NOMOGRAM and treat if above the line
- If time of ingestion unknown or patient considered unreliable, consider empiric initiation of acetylcysteine treatment
- Acetaminophen levels drawn less than 4 hr post-ingestion may be misleading.
- With the extended-release preparation, an acetaminophen level drawn less than 8 hr post-ingestion may be misleading. Draw a second level at 4–6 hr after the initial level. If either falls above the toxicity line, treatment should be initiated.
- Acetylcysteine may be withheld until acetaminophen assay results are available as long as initiation of treatment is not delayed beyond 8 hr post ingestion. If more than 8 hr post ingestion, start acetylcysteine treatment immediately.
- Loading dose: Dilute 150 mg/kg in 200 mL of 5% dextrose and administer over 30 min.
- Second dose: Dilute 50 mg/kg in 500 mL of 5% dextrose and administer over 4 hr.
- Third dose: Dilute 100 mg/kg in 1000 mL of 5% dextrose and administer over 16 hr.

IV Administration: Children
- Administer as in adults if over 40 kg
- If 20–40 kg administer
  - Loading dose: 150 mg/kg in 100 mL D_5W over 30 min
  - Second dose: 50 mg/kg in 250 mL D_5W over 4 hr
  - Third dose: 100 mg/kg in 500 mL over 16 hr
- If less than 20 kg, administer
  - Loading dose: 150 mg/kg in 3 mL/kg of D_5W over 30 min
  - Second dose: 50 mg/kg in 7 mL/kg of D_5W over 4 hr
  - Third dose: 100 mg/kg in 4 mL/kg of D_5W over 16 hr
  - Normal saline can be used if D_5W contraindicated
- Benadryl and epinephrine need to be at the bedside in case of anaphylactic reaction.
- Rate of infusion: **It is very important that NAC be given slowly.** A fast rate of infusion may cause rash, flushing, and itching. Treat with diphenhydramine and slow the infusion if symptoms occur. Please refer to the package insert for rate of infusion.
- Consult a toxicologist if giving IV NAC.

IV Administration: Children
- Administer as in adults.

Special Considerations

- Chronic ingestion of supratherapeutic doses over several hours or days
  - Evaluate for hepatotoxicity and unmetabolized acetaminophen.
  - Begin NAC if AST or ALT levels are increased and the patient has a measurable acetaminophen level.
  - Consult toxicologist for guidance on the treatment regimen.
- Late presentation: 8–24 hr postingestion
  - Evaluate for ongoing hepatotoxicity and begin NAC treatment if indicated.
  - In cases of hepatic failure, NAC has been associated with decreased cerebral edema and improved survival.
  - If patient presents close to 8 hr postingestion and it will take longer than this timeframe to obtain a level, give NAC and alter treatment as the level indicates.
  - Failure to administer NAC because of late presentation could be considered medically and legally risky.
- Extended-release acetaminophen
  - Check 4- and 8-hr acetaminophen levels and begin NAC if either level crosses the nomogram treatment line.
- Coingestants
  - Anything that delays the absorption or gastric emptying may indicate the need for more prolonged monitoring such as a large carbohydrate meal, acetaminophen mixed with an anticholinergic (e.g., diphenhydramine [Tylenol PM]), or acetaminophen and narcotic combinations.
  - Although the preceding is believed to be true, high-quality supporting research studies are not available.
- Administration of NAC and activated charcoal
  - No reason to withhold activated charcoal if a patient presents with acetaminophen overdose and is receiving oral NAC
  - No need to increase dose of NAC
- Overdose during pregnancy
  - Begin treatment as soon as possible after the overdose.
  - The fetus benefits from treatment of the mother.
- Criteria for liver transplant (King's College Hospital criteria)
  - Acetaminophen-induced (APAP) hepatotoxicity
  - pH <7.3 after adequate fluid resuscitation *or*

- Prothrombin time 100 sec or INR 6.5, *and* creatinine level >3.4 mg/dL (301 mmol/L) *plus* grade III or IV encephalopathy
- Lactate >3 mmol/L after fluid resuscitation

Admission Criteria

Admit any patient who requires NAC therapy or presents with toxic coingestants to the medical unit or to the psychiatric unit if the level is nontoxic and the patient is in danger of self-harm.

Pearls and Pitfalls

- Failure to obtain a timely acetaminophen level in the patient with an unknown or unreliable overdose can result in delayed antidote therapy.
- If the patient presents late to the ED, do not wait for the acetaminophen level before initiating treatment with the antidote.
- It is unnecessary to repeat the acetaminophen level if the first level was obtained 4 or more hours after ingestion and is above the treatment line.
- Contact hepatologist/transplant center if the following:
- Progressive coagulopathy; PT in seconds is greater than the number of hours post-ingestion (or INR >2 at 24 hr, >4 at 48 hr, or >6 at 72 hr)
- Creatinine >2.3 mg/dL (<200 mmol/L)
- Hypoglycemia
- Metabolic acidosis
- Hypotension after fluid resuscitation
- Encephalopathy

References and Suggested Readings

1. Tucker J, *www.emedicine.com/ped/topic 7.htm,* eMedicine from WebMD.
2. Acetaminophen, Micromedex™ Healthcare Series, Poisindex® vol. 128, expired June 2006.
3. Linden C, Rumack BH: Acetaminophen overdose. *Emerg Med Clin North Am* 2: 103-119, 1984.

4. Watson WA, Litovitz TL, Rodgers GC Jr, et al. 2004 Annual report of the American Association of Poison Control Centers Toxic Exposure Surveillance System. *Am J Emerg Med* 23(5):589-666, 2005.

5. Rumack BH. Acetaminophen hepatotoxicity: the first 35 years. *J Toxicol Clin Toxicol* 40(1):3-20, 2002.

Chapter 3

Antidepressants

CHANAH DeLISLE

■ Overview

Prescribed as effective treatments for illnesses such as depression and anxiety disorders and therefore readily accessible to patients at risk for suicide, antidepressant medications are the second leading cause of overdose mortality. Side effects and toxic profiles vary by class; tricyclic antidepressants (TCAs) are the most toxic. Lithium is more often used for the treatment of bipolar affective disorders, has a narrow therapeutic index and a very different presentation and management, and is addressed separately in this chapter.

1. Tricyclic Antidepressants

■ Overview

The clinician should not be reassured by a benign presentation in a patient who has potentially ingested a toxic dose of a TCA. The awake and alert patient with sinus tachycardia can become the obtunded and seizing patient with wide complex tachycardia in the time it takes to think, "Well, it's a TCA, but this patient seems stable." Tachycardia, altered mental status, or report of a possible seizure should raise the index of suspicion for TCA ingestion, as should cardiac arrest in a young, otherwise healthy person. Cardiac complications are the main cause of death in these patients.

Therapeutic uses include the following:
- Depression
- Chronic pain
- Migraine headaches
- Eating disorders
- Insomnia
- Enuresis
- Obsessive-compulsive disorders
- Anxiety disorders

Mechanisms of Action

The mechanism by which TCAs treat depression is not well understood. Other, better-understood actions of the drugs account for the dose-dependent side effects that are the identifying characteristics and complications of toxic TCA ingestions.

Substances

Cyclic Antidepressants

Amitriptyline	Desipramine	Maprotiline
Amoxapine	Doxepin	Nortriptyline
Clomipramine	Imipramine	Protriptyline
		Trimipramine

Toxicity

Without medical intervention, 15–20 mg/kg may be a lethal ingestion. It is generally stated that 10–20 mg/kg will lead to moderate or serious symptoms such as coma, and cardiovascular symptoms are expected. As little as 15 mg/kg may be fatal in a toddler.

Clinical Presentation

Remember, the drama of rapid decompensation is best avoided. When tachycardia and other anticholinergic signs and symptoms are observed, think TCA, especially if the skin is dry.

Anticholinergic Effects

- Apparent early
- Block muscarinic receptors leading to central and peripheral anticholinergic effects
- "Blind as a bat, mad as a hatter, dry as a bone, hot as a hare, red as a beet…"
- Always consider possible TCA ingestion when these effects are present (Box 3-1).

α-adrenergic Receptor Blockade Effects

Inhibits both central and peripheral α-1 and α-2 receptors, causing the following:

- Hypotension due to vasodilation.
- Reflex tachycardia.
- Miosis (possibly), therefore, mydriasis from the anticholinergic effect may not always be present with TCA overdose.

γ-Aminobutyric Acid (GABA) Antagonist Effect

- Seizure

Sodium and Potassium Channel Blockade Effects

- Sodium channel inhibition
  - QRS widening
  - PR prolongation
  - Rightward axis changes in the frontal plane
  - Right bundle branch block pattern
  - Ventricular dysrhythmias
  - Heart block and bradycardia

BOX 3-1 ▪ Antimuscarinic Toxicity	
Central Signs and Symptoms	**Peripheral Signs and Symptoms**
Delirium	Blurred vision or mydriasis
Hallucinations	Dry skin (axillae) and mouth
Myoclonus	Hyperthermia
Respiratory depression	Ileus or decreased bowel sounds
Sedation	Sinus tachycardia (most common ECG finding)
Seizures	Urinary retention
	Flushing

- Decreased myocardial contractility
- Seizures (possibly)
- Potassium channel inhibition
  - QT prolongation
  - Torsades de pointes
- Biogenic amine uptake inhibition (norepinephrine, serotonin, dopamine)
  - Tachycardia and mild hypertension
  - Myoclonus, hyperreflexia, seizures, and rigidity

Mild to Moderate Toxicity

- Central nervous system (CNS) depression and confusion
- Slurred speech and ataxia
- Dry skin (axillae) and dry mouth
- Sinus tachycardia
- Hyperreflexia

Serious Toxicity

- Coma
- Respiratory depression
- Cardiac dysrhythmia (SVT, conduction delays, ventricular dysrhythmias)
- Hypotension
- Seizures: usually generalized, single, and brief

Laboratory Evaluation

- EKG and cardiac monitoring is essential.
  - EKG findings that have been associated with TCA toxicity include:
    - R wave ≥3 mm (82% sensitivity)
    - R:S ratio >0.7 (75% sensitivity)
    - QRS >100 ms
  - Rightward axis of the terminal 40 ms of the R wave in aVR (120–270 degrees)
  - **Continuous cardiac monitoring**: obtain ECG q 2–3 hr for 6–8 hr. Monitor in ICU for 24 hr if abnormal CNS.
- Metabolic panel, ABGs, acetaminophen level (acetaminophen toxicity can be prevented if found early)
  - TCAs have more affinity for the sodium channels if acidemic, so strive to keep pH between 7.45 and 7.55.

- • TCA levels do not correspond with toxicity.
- Consider pregnancy test.

▌ Treatment

- ABCs, remembering the possibility of rapid decompensation to profound coma, seizure, and/or wide-complex tachycardias
- **Bicarb** ("amp" NaHCO$_3$ is 50 mEq) indicated for QRS > 100 ms and ventricular dysrhythmias
  - • NaHCO$_3$, 1–2 mEq/kg IV push
  - • Follow with drip, 150 mEq NaHCO$_3$ in 850-mL D$_5$W run over 4–6 hr
  - • Easily prepared by withdrawing 150 mL from a liter of D$_5$W, then adding 3 amps NaHCO$_3$
- If **seizure** requires intervention, use a benzodiazepine or barbiturate. **Do not use phenytoin.** Phenytoin also has quinidine-like properties and may worsen the cardiovascular complications of TCA toxicity. If the patient has multiple seizures, keep in mind the possibility of rhabdomyolysis.
  - • **Diazepam (Valium) 0.2–0.4 mg/kg IV up to 5–30 mg**
  - • **Lorazepam (Ativan) 0.05–0.1 mg/kg IV over 2–5 min**
  - • **Phenobarbital** 15–20 mg/kg IV
- **Hypotension**
  - • **Fluids first (LR or NS, 10–30 mL/kg)**
  - • **Norepinephrine 2 µg/min, titrate to effect**
  - • **Glucagon** 10 mg IV, then 10 mg IV over 6 hr
    - • Shown to help in some refractory cases
    - • Problem with glucagon: the hospital may not have enough to run an infusion for 6 hr.
    - • Consider glucagon as an adjunct to other pressors or with amrinone.
  - • For severe hypotension that is not responding to interventions, consider Swan-Ganz catheter or intraaortic balloon pump.
    - • Reassess, reassess, and intervene appropriately.

▌ Special Considerations

- Amoxapine: Less cardiac toxicity but can cause status epilepticus. Propofol has been suggested to terminate the seizures.
  - • **Propofol** 2.5 mg/kg IV followed by 0.2 mg/kg/min drip

Admission Criteria (Medical)

- Moderate to severe toxicity present at least 6 hr postingestion
- QRS duration greater than 100 or greater than baseline QRS
- Prolonged QTc
- History of seizure prior to arrival or abnormal level of consciousness
- Significant coingestions

Almost all patients who intentionally overdose on TCAs will need psychiatry evaluation. Accidental ingestions that are asymptomatic 6 hr postingestion may be safely discharged from the ED with close follow-up (considering living conditions, social situations, and mental capacity).

Pearls and Pitfalls

- Consider psychiatric evaluation in patients who remain free of toxic symptoms 6 hr postingestion.
- Patients with persistent signs and symptoms of overdose must be monitored continuously until all signs and symptoms have resolved.
- If the patient's baseline QRS duration is not known, monitoring should continue until it is less than 100 ms; serum level may be obtained to assist in decision-making. Subtherapeutic levels may indicate prolonged QRS is patient's baseline.
- Serotonin syndrome can occur.
- Physostigmine is not used in TCA overdose due to risk of complications associated with physostigmine (e.g., seizure, bradycardia, hypotension, asystole).
- Patient's level of consciousness can change abruptly (coma or sudden seizure).
- Never give class Ia (procainamide, disopyramide, quinidine) or Ic (flecainide, encainide, propafenone) antiarrhythmic agents. Phenytoin has similar antidysrhythmic properties.
- Sodium load hypertonic saline and alkalosis may help.

References and Suggested Readings

1. Cyclic Antidepressants. In Ellenhorn MJ, ed: *Ellenhorn's Medical Toxicology: Diagnosis and Treatment of Human Poisoning*, ed 2. Philadelphia, 1997, Lippincott Williams & Wilkins, pp 624–650.

2. Lagome E, Smollin C: Toxicity, Antidepressant. eMedicine. http://www.emedicine. com/emerg/topic37.htm. Accessed Dec 14, 2004.

3. Harrigan RA, Brady WJ: ECG abnormalities in tricyclic antidepressant overdose, *Am J Emerg Med* 17:387-393, 1999.

4. Liebelt EL, Francis PD, Woolf AD: ECG lead aVR versus QRS interval in predicting seizures and arrhythmias in acute tricyclic antidepressant toxicity, *Ann Emerg Med* 26:195-210, 1995.

5. Liebelt EL, Ulrich A, Francis PD, et al: Serial electrocardiogram changes in acute tricyclic antidepressant overdoses, *Crit Care Med* 25:1721-1726, 1997.

6. Pentel PR, Keyler DE: Cyclic Antidepressants. In Ford MD, Delaney KA, Ling LJ, Erickson T, eds: *Clinical Toxicology*. Philadelphia, 2001, WB Saunders.

7. Sarko J: Antidepressant, old and new, *Emerg Med Clin North Am* 18:637–654, 2000.

8. Weisman RS, Howland MA, Hoffman RS, et al: *Goldfrank's toxicologic emergencies*, ed 5. Norwalk, CT, 1994, Appleton and Lange, pp 725-733.

9. Wolfe TR, Caravati EM, Rollins DE: Terminal 40-ms frontal plane QRS axis as a marker for tricyclic antidepressant overdose, *Ann Emerg Med* 18:348-351, 1989.

2. Selective Serotonin Reuptake Inhibitors

Overview

Selective serotonin reuptake inhibitors (SSRIs) have become the first line of treatment of depression. These newer antidepressants have far fewer side effects than predecessors and are less toxic in overdose. Therapeutic uses include management of depression, obsessive-compulsive disorders, smoking cessation, obesity, eating disorders, and alcoholism.

Substances

- SSRI: fluoxetine, fluvoxamine, paroxetine, sertraline, citalopram
- SSRI + alpha antagonist: trazodone, nefazodone
- SSRI + inhibit reuptake of NE and dopamine: venlafaxine
- α-2 antagonist: mirtazapine
- Inhibit reuptake of biogenic amines: bupropion

Toxicity

Compared with TCAs, these agents are typically well tolerated in overdose. However, it is the dose that makes the poison.

- Fluoxetine: Adults that ingest more than 900 mg may develop seizures.
- Paroxetine: Generally well tolerated in overdose scenarios. Adults that ingest more than 3600 mg may develop serotonin syndrome (see below).
- Sertraline: Ingestion of more than 2 g in an adult may produce serotonin syndrome or even death (in a person who reportedly took 2.5 g).
- Fluvoxamine: Death is rare. Ingestion of more than 1.5 g may cause severe CNS depression (i.e., coma), bradycardia, or nothing at all.
- Citalopram: Overdoses of more than 600 mg may lead to seizures and EKG changes (QTc prolongation, sinus tachycardia, widened QRS).
- Bupropion has caused seizures in slightly-higher-than-therapeutic doses.

Clinical Presentation

- Patient will typically present with tachycardia, dizziness, nausea and vomiting, fatigue or agitation, or tremor.
- Occasionally CNS depression is present. Although seizures rarely occur, they may present early.
- Fatalities have been reported but are generally related to multiple drug ingestions.
- EKG changes such as sinus tachycardia, QRS widening, and QTc prolongation may be seen in significant citalopram overdoses.
- Serotonin syndrome (see below)

Serotonin Syndrome

Serotonin syndrome (SS) has a mortality rate of 11%–15% if not treated (not necessarily in overdose). SS can be precipitated by drug-drug interaction, single dose, or high therapeutic doses of serotonergic medications and not necessarily in overdose. Remember, SS has been reported with single drug use as well. SS is a clinical diagnosis made when, in the absence of a neuroleptic or a drug whose toxic profile would explain the symptoms, three of the following are present:

- Altered mental status (including hypomania and confusion)
- Hyperreflexia

- Agitation
- Myoclonus
- Diaphoresis
- Tremor or shivering
- Diarrhea
- Lack of coordination
- Hyperpyrexia (Remember to obtain the **appropriate** core temperature; avoid obtaining the tympanic or axillary temperature.)

Severe cases can proceed to rhabdomyolysis, renal failure, coagulopathy and disseminated intravascular coagulation (DIC), autonomic instability, and status epilepticus.

Differential Diagnosis

Consider anticholinergic or sympathomimetic poisoning, aspirin toxicity, withdrawal syndromes (alcohol, barbiturates, and other sedative hypnotics), neuroleptic malignant syndrome, hyperthyroidism, or infection.

Laboratory Evaluation

- EKG
    - Citalopram has been reported to cause seizures and widening of the QRS. Seizures may occur early. EKG changes may occur as late as 24 hr after ingestion.
    - Fluvoxamine may present with bradycardia.
- Monitor for CNS depression and seizures.
- Chemistry panel, acetaminophen
    - Acetaminophen is readily available and can be a killer if the antidote is not given in time (see Chapter 2).
- Consider pregnancy test.
- Creatine kinase (CK) (consider rhabdomyolysis, especially with "tea-colored" urine and elevated K).

Treatment

- Provide supportive care.
- Address ABCs.

- If mental status is altered or seizing, consider SNOT (sugar, naloxone, oxygen, thiamine).
- Treat **seizure** with benzodiazepines and barbiturates.
  - **Valium** 0.2–0.4 mg/kg IV up to 5–30 mg
  - **Ativan** 0.05–0.1 mg/kg IV over 2–5 min
  - **Phenobarbital** 15–20 mg/kg IV
- Treat **prolonged QRS** with bicarb.
- $NaHCO_3$, 1–2 mEq/kg IV push
- Follow with drip, 150 mEq $NaHCO_3$ in 850-mL D_5W run over 4–6 hr.
- Easily prepared by withdrawing 150 mL from a liter of D_5W, then adding 3 amps $NaHCO_3$
- Hyperpyrexia (likely due to muscle rigidity)
- External cooling
- Benzodiazepines
  - **Valium** 0.2–0.4 mg/kg IV up to 5–30 mg
  - **Ativan** 0.05–0.1 mg/kg IV over 2–5 min
  - **Clonazepam** may help control myoclonus
- Use nondepolarizing paralysis if necessary.
- Rhabdomyolysis
  - 150 mEq $NaHCO_3$ in 850-mL D_5W at 150–250 mL/hr

Special Considerations

- Overdose
  - A combination of drugs is not necessary to cause SS. A single acute ingestion is enough.

Admission Criteria

- Overdose
- Abnormal vital signs, especially temperature elevation
- Seizure prior to arrival or in ED
- Altered mental status after appropriate period of observation in ED
- EKG abnormalities such as the following:
  - Prolonged QTc, especially if greater that 450 ms
  - Sinus tachycardia greater than 110
  - Dysrhythmias

Pearls and Pitfalls

- Besides the usual serotonergic culprit drugs involved in serotonin syndrome, consider St. John's Wort, meperidine (Demerol), dextromethorphan, cocaine, tramadol, lithium, and ecstasy.
- Perform continuous EEG monitoring if seizures are a problem and patient requires nondepolarizing paralysis.
- Consider rhabdomyolysis.
- Serotonin syndrome generally resolves within 24 hr after removing the inciting agent but can last for several days.

References and Suggested Readings

1. LoCurto MJ: The serotonin syndrome, *Emer Med Clin North Am* 15:665-675, 1997.
2. Sarko J: Antidepressant, old and new, *Emerg Med Clin North Am* 18:637-654, 2000.
3. Stork CM: Serotonin reuptake inhibitor and a typical antidepressants. In Goldfrank LR, Flomenbaum N, Lewin N, et al., eds: *Goldfrank's toxicologic emergencies*, ed. New York, 2002, McGraw-H:11.
4. Arnold DH: The central serotonin syndrome: paradigm for psychotherapeutic misadventure, *Pediatr Rev* 23:427-432, 2002.

3. Lithium

Overview

- Therapeutic levels: 0.6–1.2 mEq/L
- Narrow therapeutic index
- Rapid absorption of therapeutic dose
  - Peak levels at 2–4 hr after ingestion, complete absorption at 8 hr
  - Levels in overdose may not peak until 72 hr.
- Volume of distribution: 0.6–0.9 L/kg
- 95% of lithium is excreted by the kidney, dependent on glomerular filtration rate (GFR)
- Half-life: 20–24 hr, with elimination half-life up to 58 hr in older adults
- Mechanism of action is unknown, but lithium enters cells via active transport.
- Used in industry for batteries and nuclear reactor coolant; occupational toxicity is rare.

Therapeutic Uses

- Bipolar affective disorders
- Cluster headaches
- Cell stimulation (chemotherapy-induced neutropenia)

Substances

Lithium carbonate	Lithobid	Eskalith

Toxicity

- Toxic symptoms do not correlate with blood levels.
- Prolonged exposure of the central nervous system (CNS) to toxic lithium levels can cause permanent sequelae.
- Toxicity may be acute or chronic, or acute **on** chronic (over-dose by current lithium user).
- Acute toxicity is typically seen in those naive to lithium use.
  - Accidental ingestion by a child
  - Adult taking someone else's pills
- Chronic toxicity may be precipitated by:
  - Increase in dosage
  - Dosage error
  - Renal dysfunction
  - Dehydration
  - Illness
  - Other medications
  - Alterations in sodium or potassium
  - Risk of dehydration and retention of sodium and lithium outweighs the possible benefit of small increase in excretion.

Clinical Presentation

- See Table 3-1
- Hyperthermia is a bad prognostic indicator; it may be connected with neuroleptic malignant syndrome (NMS) or serotonin syndrome.
- Patients who are already taking lithium chronically and then take an acute overdose may present differently (acute on chronic toxicity).
  - Signs and symptoms of both acute and chronic toxicity present

Table 3-1 ACUTE AND CHRONIC TOXICITY OF LITHIUM

		Acute	Chronic
Gastrointestinal		Nausea	Minimal if any
		Vomiting	
		Diarrhea	
Cardiovascular		Orthostatic hypotension	Myocarditis
		Nonspecific ST, T wave changes	
		Prolonged QT interval	
		Rare malignant dysrhythmias	
Neurologic	Mild	Fine tremors of hands	Similar
		Dizziness, lightheadedness	
		Weakness	
	Moderate	Agitation, apathy, drowsiness	Similar
		Fasciculations	
		Tinnitus	
		Slurred speech	
		Hyperreflexia	
	Severe	Altered mental status	Memory deficits
		Confusion	Severe Parkinson's disease
		Lethargy	Psychosis
		Coma	Pseudotumor cerebri
		Clonus	
		Choreoathetosis	
		Seizures	
Renal		Concentrating defects	Nephrogenic diabetes insipidus
			Interstitial nephritis
Hematologic		Leukocytosis	Aplastic anemia
Endocrine		None	Hypothyroidism
Dermatologic		None	Ulcers
			Dermatitis
			Localized edema

- Patient may seem well, then suddenly decompensate
- Increased half-life because of chronic usage, therefore more severe toxicity than acute

▌ Laboratory Evaluation

- Obtain lithium level, electrolytes, and acetaminophen level if coingestion is suspected. If hypernatremia, think nephrogenic diabetes insipidus, especially with polyuria.

- Repeat lithium level in 2 hr for acute ingestion, *or 6–12 hr in chronic toxicity for 24 hr, then daily.*
- Monitor fluid and electrolytes (chemistry panel). Pay close attention to sodium and potassium levels. Lithium looks like sodium and potassium to the cell; it has the same valences as the common ions.
  - Low sodium potentiates a high intracellular lithium level.
  - Renal function, GFR (sometimes estimated on the UA). UA can be used to quickly assess the patient's fluid status.
- EKG: Significant toxicity can lead to blocks, sinus node dysfunction and bradycardia, and prolonged QTc.
- Consider thyroid function testing.
- Fluid input and urine output (urinary catheter may be necessary). If polyuria, think nephrogenic diabetes insipidus.

Treatment

- Address basics: airway, breathing, circulation.
- IV of 0.9% saline
  - Maintain circulating volume to promote urine output.
  - Forced diuresis has not been shown to increase lithium clearance. However, 0.9% saline at a rate of 150- to 300-mL/hr for several hours is appropriate for patients with impaired glomerular filtration rate.
  - No role for diuretics
    - Lithium toxicity increases with salt and water depletion.
    - Do not use osmotic diuretics, phosphodiesterase inhibitors, or carbonic anhydrase inhibitors.

Activated Charcoal

- Administer for possible coingestions.
- Activated charcoal does not adsorb lithium.

Whole Bowel Irrigation

- Administer polyethylene glycol (PEG-ES) PO or NG.
  - 2 L/hr until effluent clear (500 mL/hr for children)
  - Enhances GI clearance
  - Important for sustained release preparations
  - Monitor fluid and electrolyte status closely, although these are not major risks.

Hemodialysis

- Indications
  - Renal failure
  - Altered mental status
  - Severe neurologic dysfunction
  - Stable but preexisting condition limiting IV fluids (congestive heart failure, pulmonary edema)
  - High serum levels of lithium (Table 3-2)
- **Do not remove dialysis catheter until confident that lithium level will not rebound with redistribution of the drug.** Lithium levels can rise for as long as 4 days after admission. Repeat level 6 hr after end of dialysis.
- Hemodialysis clears lithium at a rate of 70–170 mL/min; healthy kidneys clear at a rate of 10–40 mL/min; peritoneal dialysis (PD) is less efficacious than healthy kidneys, clearing at a rate of 10–15 mL/min.
- Peritoneal dialysis would be initially helpful in a patient with renal failure and a PD catheter that is already placed. Keep in mind that this patient may require hemodialysis.

Special Considerations

- Lithium is highly concentrated in the thyroid gland.
  - Lithium toxicity can exacerbate hypothyroidism to the degree of myxedema coma.
- Drug–drug interactions
  - Drugs that increase lithium levels: thiazide diuretics, ACE inhibitors, NSAIDS (except aspirin)
  - Drugs that decrease lithium levels: methylxanthines, loop, osmotic and potassium-sparing diuretics, acetazolamide

Table 3-2 INDICATIONS FOR HEMODIALYSIS

Lithium Level	Indications for Dialysis
<2.5 mEq/L	End-stage renal disease
2.5–4 mEq/L	Acute or chronic ingestion
	Severe neurologic symptoms
	Hemodynamic instability
	Renal insufficiency/ESRD
>4 mEq/L	All of the above
	Acute igestion

Admission Criteria

- AMS, including confusion
  - Order fall precautions. Suicide patients will need one-to-one watch while on medicine ward to prevent further attempts at suicide.
- Ataxic and vulnerable patients
  - Make sure fall precautions are ordered.
- Dehydrated and compromised renal function
- Cardiovascular abnormality: bradycardia, hypotension
  - Monitored bed
- Significant coingestions
- Indications for dialysis

Pearls and Pitfalls

- Lithium levels in chronic toxicity may be high normal or slightly above normal.
- Lithium may cause sinus node dysfunction and bradycardia.
- Nephrology Service should be notified early in cases of significant lithium toxicity.
- Lithium-toxic patients with renal insufficiency will not be able to excrete lithium sufficiently and may deteriorate rapidly.
- Check thyroid function.
- CNS symptoms predominate in both acute and chronic toxicity.
- Think coingestants, especially in acute overdose situations.

References and Suggested Readings

1. Ellenhorn MJ, Schonwald S, Ordog G, et al: Lithium. In Ellenhorn MJ, Schonwald S, Ordog G, eds: *Medical toxicology: diagnosis and treatment of human poisoning*, Baltimore, 1997, Williams and Wilkins.
2. Henry GC: Lithium. In Goldfrank LR, Flomenbaum NE, Lewin NA, et al, eds: *Toxicologic emergencies*, ed 6, Stamford, CT, 1998, Appleton and Lange.
3. Timmer RT, Sands JM: Lithium intoxication, *J Amer Soc Nephrol* 10:666-675, 1999.

Chapter 4

Benzodiazepines

JOEL S. HOLGER

Overview

Benzodiazepines cause toxicity via their interaction with the γ-aminobutyric acid (GABA) system. Tolerance to benzodiazepines is common. Abrupt discontinuation of long-term use will precipitate a potentially lethal withdrawal syndrome. **Pure benzodiazepine overdose is very lethal**. Patients at risk for adverse outcome include the following:

- Older adults
- Alcohol or other depressant drug coingestions
- Prolonged immobilization (rhabdomyolysis)

See substances list on following page.

Toxicity

- **Most common toxic effects** are ataxia, lethargy, and slurred speech.
- The **most feared toxicity** is respiratory depression.
- Severe central nervous system (CNS) depression (i.e., coma) is rare and usually occurs with another coingestion, especially alcohol.
- Short-acting agents such as temazepam, alprazolam, and triazolam may be more toxic. The reason is likely due to increased respiratory depression, but these agents also may be more likely to be abused and mixed with alcohol.

Substances

Diazepam (Valium)

Lorazepam (Ativan)

Midazolam (Versed)

Chlordiazepoxide (Librium)

Clonazepam (Klonopin)

Temazepam (Restoril)

Triazolam (Halcion)

Flurazepam (Dalmane)

Alprazolam (Xanax)

Oxazepam (Serax)

Flunitrazepam (Rohypnol)

_____

The brand name is indicated in parentheses.

Clinical Presentation

The vast majority of patients demonstrate sedation consistent with the sedative-hypnotic toxidrome (see Tox Mnemonics section).
- Other clinical effects in overdose may include hypothermia, hypotension, and bradycardia.
- The pupils are usually unaffected, but miosis or mydriasis may occur. Nystagmus has been described.
- Clinical suspicion is most valuable.
- Tolerance to benzodiazepines is common.
- Abrupt discontinuation of long-term use will precipitate a potentially lethal withdrawal syndrome.

Laboratory Evaluation

- Blood levels or other blood tests are not helpful.
- Urine assays may be helpful but are insensitive if the benzodiazepine does not have the oxazepam metabolite, especially clonazepam (Klonopin) and lorazepam (ativan).

- Consider acetaminophen level in case of coingestion.
- It is important to monitor vital signs and level of consciousness in patients with coingestions of CNS depressants (including ethanol).

Treatment

- Airway protection if the patient demonstrates significant respiratory depression or coma
- Activated charcoal (1 g/kg) if the patient presents within 60 min postingestion of a potentially toxic amount of the benzodiazepine
- General supportive care
- Diuresis and hemodialysis are ineffective.
- **Flumazenil**
  - Flumazenil is a specific antidote for benzodiazepine toxicity. It is a competitive antagonist at the benzodiazepine receptor.
  - Effects are dose-related; most patients respond to a total dose of 1 mg IV.
  - Flumazenil does not consistently fully reverse respiratory depression.
  - The reversal effect lasts from 45–60 min; resedation may occur at 20–120 min.
  - Flumazenil may have a role in reversing the well-defined pure benzodiazepine overdose in a nonchronic user without a seizure disorder. These patients are rare. *The accidental ingestion in a pediatric patient may fit this scenario.*
  - Contraindications to flumazenil use include the following:
    - Underlying seizure disorder (use of flumazenil may precipitate or unmask seizures)
    - Chronic use of or dependence on benzodiazepine (use of flumazenil may precipitate acute benzodiazepine withdrawal or seizures)
    - Coingestion of tricyclic antidepressants (TCAs) or any drug known to be proconvulsive (i.e., causing seizures) in overdose, such as cocaine or theophylline. Flumazenil may precipitate seizures in these patients.
    - Closed head injury (another seizure precaution)
    - **Remember, use of flumazenil may unmask the toxic effects of coingested drugs** (many of which are unknown in the clinical scenario).

- Procedure for flumazenil use:
  - The patient must have CNS depression and normal vital signs. In other words, the patient should be symptomatic.
  - The patient has a normal ECG (to help rule out TCA ingestion) and nonfocal deficit neurological exam.
  - Use slow IV titration of 0.1 mg/min to a total dose of 1.0 mg.
  - After this, a continuous infusion of 0.25–1.0 mg/hr in saline may be used (not FDA approved) or re-bolusing if sedation reoccurs.

There is no evidence that the use of flumazenil improves outcome when compared with standard supportive care.

Special Considerations

- Paradoxical reactions can occur with triazolam (Halcion, Upjohn, Kalamazoo, MI) and flurazepam (Dalmane Roche Labs, Nutely, NJ).
- Abrupt discontinuation of long-term use will precipitate a potentially lethal withdrawal syndrome.
- Short-acting agents such as temazepam, alprazolam, and triazolam may be more toxic. The reason is likely due to increased respiratory depression, but they also may be more likely to be abused and mixed with alcohol.

Admission Criteria

- Signs or symptoms of CNS sedation
- Coingestants
- Patients treated with flumazenil
- Patients observed for 4-6 hr without signs of CNS toxicity may be discharged from the ED.

Pearls and Pitfalls

- Clinical suspicion is valuable.
- Beware of the patient who coingests benzodiazepines with sedatives, especially narcotics or alcohol.
- Resedation is common after successful flumazenil reversal.
- Flumazenil should be rarely used in acute overdose situations.

References and Suggested Readings

1. Goldfrank LR: Flumazenil: a pharmacologic antidote with limited medical toxicology utility, or... an antidote in search of an overdose? *Acad Emerg Med* 4:935-936, 1997.

2. Mathieu-Nolf M, Babe MA, Coquelle-Couplet V, et al: Flumazenil use in an emergency department: a survey, *J Toxicol Clin Toxicol* 39:15-20, 2001.

3. Osborn HH: Sedative-hypnotic agents. In Goldfrank LR, Flomenbaum NE, Lewin NA, et al, eds: *Goldfrank's toxicologic emergencies,* ed 6, Stamford, CT, 1998, Appleton and Lange, pp 1001-1022.

4. Wiley CC, Wiley JF Jr: Pediatric benzodiazepine ingestion resulting in hospitalization, *J Toxicol Clin Toxicol* 36:227-231, 1998.

Chapter 5

Atypical Antipsychotics

KATHLEEN A. NEACY AND CARSON R. HARRIS

Overview

Atypical antipsychotics ("the second generation") have been introduced to the U.S. market within the last 20 years as replacements for traditional antipsychotics such as thioridazine, haloperidol, perphenazine, and chlorpromazine. They are indicated for the management of schizophrenia, especially negative (deficit) symptoms of schizophrenia (e.g., flat affect, social withdrawal), obsessive-compulsive disorder (OCD), refractory psychoses, mood disorders, and some cases of borderline personality disorder. Atypical antipsychotics are more selective D_2 antagonists with highest affinity in the mesolimbic receptors. In 2004, the AAPCC Poison Center reported 38,315 atypical antipsychotic ingestions, 2098 with serious effects and 94 deaths. Overdoses are commonly seen with multiple coingestants, but outcomes are typically good.

Substances

Clozapine (1990)	Risperidone (1993)
Olanzapine (1996)	Quetiapine (1997)
Ziprasidone (2001)	Aripiprazole (2002)

The parenthetical number refers to the year in which the drug was introduced to the U.S. market.

Toxicity

- Inhibit 5HT$_{2A}$ receptors to greater extent than dopaminergic receptors.
- In general, they have minimal to no extrapyramidal effects.
- Combination with other drugs that involve CYP450 system in their metabolism (Table 5-1) may increase toxicity.
- **Aripiprazole** daily dose is 10–30 mg/day.

			Mechanism of Action		
Substance	**H$_1$**	**α$_1$**	**α$_2$**	**M1**	**5HT$_{2A}$**
Clozapine	3+	3+	3+	4+	3+
Risperidone	-	2+	1+	-	3+
Olanzapine	2+	2+	-	3+	3+
Quetiapine	3+	3+	-	3+	2+
Ziprasidone	-	3+	-	-	3+
Aripiprazole	-	2+	-	-	2+*

Aripiprazole has partial D$_2$ agonist (presynaptically) and regulates partial agonist 5HT$_{1A}$.

Clinical Presentation

See Box 5-1.

QT Prolongation

- All atypical antipsychotics can cause QT prolongation.
  - QT prolongation may present as syncope or ventricular arrhythmias, including torsades de pointes.

Table 5-1 Atypical Antipsychotics Metabolism and Dosing			
Substance	**CYP450 Isoenzymes**	**Daily Dose (mg)**	**Half-life (hr)**
Clozapine	1A2, 2D6, 3A4, 2C9, 2C19	100–900	10–105
Risperidone	2D6, 3A4?	4–16*	3–24
Olanzapine	1A2, 2C19, 2D6	5–20	20–70
Quetiapine	3A4, 2D6	150–800	4–10
Ziprasidone	3A4	60–160	4–10

Patients taking >6 mg/day have a greater risk of developing EPS.

> **BOX 5-1 ▪ COMMON SIDE EFFECTS FROM ROUTINE (PRESCRIBED) USE OF ATYPICAL ANTIPSYCHOTICS**
>
> Metabolic disturbances, hyperglycemia
>
> Dyslipidemia especially increased triglyceridemia
>
> Hyperprolactinemia especially with risperidone
>
> QT prolongation
>
> May precipitate diabetes; DKA (rarely)
>
> Weight gain (occasionally)
>
> Amenorrhea, galactorrhea, gynecomastia

- Involves blockade of the potassium rectifier channel (I_{rK}) (Table 5-2)
- Malignant arrhythmias related to treatment with atypical antipsychotics are extremely rare. One reported case involved a patient with ventricular tachycardia who had underlying myocardial ischemia and concurrent treatment with **clozapine**.
- **Quetiapine** is associated with QT prolongation when used concurrently with other P450 inhibitors.
- Prospective studies of QT prolongation by atypical antipsychotics are limited and ongoing.

Withdrawal States

Reports of symptoms following discontinuation of medication include:

- Panic attacks
- Rebound anxiety
- Flulike symptoms
- Somatic complaints, especially nausea, headache, and diarrhea; may include tachycardia, gait instability, or tremor
- Delirium has been associated with abrupt discontinuation of clozapine.

Table 5-2 DEGREE OF QT PROLONGATION

Substance	QT Prolongation (msec) (Range)
Ziprasidone	20 (6–10*)
Quetiapine	14 (9.5–16.5)
Risperidone	11 (7.4–15.8)
Olanzapine	7

*From www.torsades.org, accessed Apr 1, 2005.

- If clozapine needs to be discontinued (e.g., for agranulocytosis), an anticholinergic agent combined with a traditional antipsychotic such as thioridazine can help ameliorate withdrawal symptoms.

Overdose

See Table 5-3.

- Very little information on **aripiprazole** overdose (OD) is available, but vomiting, tachycardia, and somnolence have been reported to date.
- **Clozapine** has been associated with **respiratory depression** when there is a benzodiazepine coingestion.
  - Because of the need for weekly or biweekly blood tests and the fact that patients are only given a week's supply of medication, OD is unusual unless the patient is "hoarding."
  - Infrequent complications of clozapine OD: fasciculations, rotational nystagmus, T-wave flattening on EKG
- *Some side effects may be exacerbated in OD.*
  - Reports of mania induced by olanzapine in HIV seropositive patients with schizophrenia

Table 5-3 OVERDOSE TOXICITY

Symptoms	Clozapine	Risperidone	Quetiapine	Olanzapine	Ziprasidone
Lethargy	42%	50%	47%	76%	
Coma	42%			28%	
Confusion	20%			38%	
Agitation	18%		7%	33%	
Dysarthria				28%	Yes
Vomiting/diarrhea					Yes
Urinary retention					Yes
Miosis				38%	
Anticholinergic	20%			43%	
Widened QRS		4%		Yes	
Long QTc	Yes	10%		Yes	Yes
ST changes				14%	
Tachycardia	39%	31%	27%	52%	
Hypotension	10%	12%	6%		
Hypertension		23%		19%	
Myoclonus				24%	
Seizure	10%		1%		
Death	10%	2%	0%	No	No

- One reported case of *elevated temperature* and elevated creatine kinase in **olanzapine** OD; did not meet criteria for neuroleptic malignant syndrome
- The maximal overdose of **quetiapine** reported to manufacturers is 9600 mg, and there was an associated hypokalemia and first-degree heart block.
- Coingestion of benzodiazepines worsens hypotension.
- **Risperidone** and coingestion of SSRI, benzodiazepine, or tricyclic antidepressants (TCA) has been reported to cause seizure or coma.
  - 1 fatality due to risperidone OD and coingestion of TCA
  - Risperidone has a high affinity for α-adrenergic receptors and therefore may lead to hypotension and tachycardia.

Laboratory Evaluation

- EKG and check for
  - QT prolongation, sinus tachycardia, ventricular dysrhythmias (infrequent)
- Laboratory studies
  - CBC, electrolytes; urine toxicology panel, ASA and/or acetaminophen if coingestions suspected
  - Liver function tests
- Antipsychotic drug levels are probably not helpful in emergency management but may be obtained if the clinician wishes to follow serial levels for admitted patients. Remember, the results will take several days in most institutions.
  - Patients on chronic meds will tolerate higher serum levels.
  - It is difficult to correlate serum levels with OD symptoms.
  - Hepatic insufficiency if decreased P450 metabolism suspected

Treatment

- Management of known or suspected atypical antidepressant overdose
  - Airway as needed because decreased mental status is common and aspiration risk is high
  - Breathing
  - Circulation
    - Hypotension (common) or circulatory collapse (infrequent) associated with OD

- Atypical antipsychotics have a high binding affinity for α-adrenergic receptors, resulting in hypotension and tachycardia.
- Avoid epinephrine and dopamine for pressure support. Use an α-receptor agonist for pressure support: phenylephrine, levarterenol, or metaraminol.
- Avoid type 1a antidysrhythmic agents (per the Clozaril package insert [Novartis Pharmaceuticals, East Hanover, NJ]; not supported in the literature).
- Other adjuncts
  - Physostigmine may ameliorate clozapine-induced delirium.
    - May also exacerbate hypersalivation and epileptogenic potential
    - Reverses peripheral and central anticholinergic symptoms
    - Do not use if EKG changes present.
  - Use caution in treating agitation with benzodiazepines, which may exacerbate hypotension.
- Decontamination
  - Use single-dose activated charcoal; use of multiple-dose activated charcoal not supported in literature
  - Hemodialysis: rarely indicated
    - Atypical antipsychotics are highly protein bound and thus hemodialysis will likely be ineffective in clearing the drug.

▉ Special Considerations

Duration of EKG monitoring required in OD is unclear.

- For nonsustained release preparations, the standard 6-hr observation is prudent, but currently no prospective studies exist to clearly define observation standards.
- Repeat EKG at 6 hr; if negative, patient may be clinically cleared.

▉ Admission Criteria

- Intensive care unit admission for hypotension, compromised airway, or mental status changes
- Admit to a monitored bed for EKG changes in hemodynamically stable patients

- Psychiatric consultation as needed for dosing changes, acute withdrawal symptoms, or assessment of suicide risk

Pearls and Pitfalls

- Atypical antipsychotics are extremely safe in routine use.
- Overdoses of atypical antipsychotics are rarely fatal.
- Most common symptoms of overdose include mental status changes, tachycardia, and hypotension. Supportive care is usually adequate.
- Coingestion of benzodiazepines, TCAs, and occasionally SSRIs can worsen hemodynamic compromise in OD.
- Usual supportive care for OD patients is indicated: decontamination, screening laboratory studies, EKG, and psychiatric consultation.

References and Suggested Readings

1. Atypical neuroleptics. In Poisindex® System. [Intranot database]. Version 5.1. Greenwood Village, Colo: Thomson Micromedex.
2. Burns MJ: The pharmacology and toxicology of atypical antipsychotic agents, *J Toxicol Clin Toxicol* 39:1-14, 2001.
3. Cohen LG Fatalo A, Thompson BT, et al: Olanzapine overdose with serum concentrations, *Ann Emerg Med* 34:275-278, 1999.
4. Glassman AH, Bigger JT: Antipsychotic drugs: prolonged QTc interval, torsades de pointes, and sudden death, *Am J Psychiatry* 158:1774-1782, 2001.
5. Goldberg JF: Psychiatric emergencies: new drugs in psychiatry, *Emerg Med Clin North Am* 18:211–231, 2000.
6. Kopala LC, Day C, Dillman B, et al: A case of risperidone overdose in early schizophrenia: a review of potential complications, *J Psychiat Neurosci* 23:305–308, 1998.
7. Mahoney MC, Connolly BF, Smith CM, et al: A clozapine overdose with markedly elevated serum levels, *J Clin Pharm* 39:97-100, 1999.
8. Trenton A: Fatalities associated with therapeutic use and OD of atypical antipsychotics. *CNS Drugs* 17:307-324, 2003.
9. Watson WA, Livovitz TL, Rodgers GC, et al: 2004. Report of the American Association of Poison Control Centers toxic exposure surveillance system, *Am J Emerg Med* 23:589–666, 2005.
10. Welber MR, Nevins S: Clozapine overdose: a case report, *J Emerg Med* 13:199-202, 1995.
11. Wirshing DA, Pierre JM, Erhart SM, Boyd JA: Understanding the new and evolving profile of adverse drug effects in schizophrenia, *Psychiatr Clin North Am* 26:165-190, 2003.

Chapter 6

Antihistamines and Anticholinergics

Joel S. Holger

▌ Overview

Antihistamines and anticholinergics are widely available and usually do not require prescriptions. They are most commonly used to relieve cold and allergy symptoms. Patients who use these medications can usually be identified from the history; however, the pattern of the specific toxidrome may be required to recognize toxicity in the patient. Intentional abuse (e.g., of jimsonweed) may be seen.

▌ Substances

First-Generation Anticholinergics	Second-Generation Anticholinergics (Nonsedating, Primarily H-1 Blockers, with Little Anticholinergic Effect)
Chlorpheniramine	Cetirizine
Cyproheptadine	Desloratadine
Dimenhydrinate	Fexofenadine
Diphenhydramine	Loratidine
Doxylamine	
Hydroxyzine	
Jimsonweed	

Toxicity

- The toxic effects of antihistamines are manifested by their interaction with H-1 or H-2 receptors.
- The toxic effects of anticholinergics are manifested by their interaction with acetylcholine receptors, which may be divided into the following:
  - Muscarinic (e.g., mydriasis, dry skin and mouth, urinary retention, or decreased gut motility)
  - Nicotinic (muscle weakness)
  - Central nervous system (CNS) (e.g., anxiety, confusion, ataxia, hallucinations, sedation, coma, or seizures). Sedation is most common.
- Antihistamines have an affinity to interact with cholinergic receptors and cause *anticholinergic syndrome*.
- The newer, "second-generation" nonsedating antihistamines have low affinity for cholinergic receptors and low penetration into the CNS. These predominantly cause cardiac dysrhythmias in toxicity (i.e., torsades de pointes).
- H-2 receptor medication toxicity
  - Toxic effects of these medications are rare.

Clinical Presentation

Anticholinergic Syndrome

- A combination of peripheral and central toxic effects:
  - "*Mad as a hatter* (delirium), *red as a beet* (skin vasodilatation, **flushing**), *dry as a bone* (dry skin and mouth), *hot as Hades* (hyperthermia), and *blind as a bat* (loss of accommodation, **mydriasis**)."
- Tachycardia is a consistent finding (QRS and QT prolongation may occur), hence, "tacky as a polyester suit."

Laboratory Evaluation

There are no laboratory findings that distinguish the toxicity of these agents from other toxicities.

- Monitor vital signs for hypertension, hyperthermia, tachycardia, and dysrhythmias.
- Creatine kinase (CPK) for development of rhabdomyolysis, urine assay for blood (myoglobin can be qualitatively positive for blood).

Treatment

Anticholinergic Syndrome

- Cardiac monitor
- Activated charcoal (1 g/kg) if given within 1 hr of ingestion
- IV fluids (normal saline for hypotension), and use vasopressors (dopamine) if unresponsive to fluids
- Benzodiazepines if seizures occur
- Esmolol if tachycardic with evidence of ischemia (0.5 µg/kg IV over 1 min, 50 µg/kg/min drip and titrate)
- Consider physostigmine.
  - Physostigmine is a short-acting acetylcholinesterase inhibitor that prevents the breakdown of acetylcholine at the synapse. In this syndrome, the muscarinic end organ effects are reversed. Physostigmine increases vagal tone at the heart, decreasing the heart rate. As a tertiary amine, it crosses the blood-brain barrier and reverses the CNS effects of toxicity. Torsades de pointes is not reversed in nonsedating antihistamine toxicity.

When to Use Physostigmine
- Ingestion of an anticholinergic agent is strongly suspected and toxic manifestations are severe enough to warrant reversal.
- Agitation, delirium, seizures, coma

Dosing Guidelines for Physostigmine
- Adults: 1 mg slow IV push (over 3–5 min), repeat every 10 min to effect (up to 4 mg)
- Children: 0.02 mg/kg over 5 min
- Repeat doses may be required every 30–60 min.

Physostigmine Observation Points
- Seizures
- Bradycardia
  - Atropine (at half the regular dose of physostigmine) may be used if bradycardia occurs.
- Patients who have been given physostigmine should be admitted to a monitored bed for further observation.

When Not to Use Physostigmine
- Presence of tricyclic antidepressants or Class Ia or Ic medications
- Conduction defects and AV block
- Relative: bronchospastic disease

- **Using physostigmine in the presence of tricyclic antidepressant medications may precipitate asystole.**

Torsades de pointes

- Cardioversion followed by
- Magnesium sulfate (2–6 g in adults, 25–50 mg/kg in children) over 15 to 30 min
- Overdrive pacing may be required.

Admission Criteria

- Use of physostigmine
- Significant tachycardia and QRS/QTc prolongation
- Agitation
- Moderate to severe sedation
- Seizures
- Torsades de pointes

Pearls and Pitfalls

- Not recognizing the ingestion of tricyclic antidepressants.
- Not recognizing bladder distention or Foley catheter placement.
- Administering physostigmine rapidly (seizures may occur).
- These overdoses may cause an ileus, resulting in delayed absorption.

References and Suggested Readings

1. Burns MJ, Linden CH, Graudins A, et al: A comparison of physostigmine and benzodiazepines for the treatment of anticholinergic poisoning, *Ann Emerg Care* 37:239-241, 2001.
2. Koppel C, Ibe K, Tenczer J: Clinical symptomatology of diphenhydramine overdose: an evaluation of 130 cases, 1982 to 1985, *J Toxicol Clin Toxicol* 25:53-70, 1987.
3. Pentel P, Peterson CD: Asystole complicating physostigmine treatment of tricyclic antidepressant overdose, *Ann Emerg Med* 9:588-590, 1980.
4. Shannon M: Toxicology reviews: physostigmine, *Pediatr Emerg Care* 14:224-226, 1998.
5. Weisman RS: Antihistamines and decongestants. In Goldfrank LR, Flomenbaum NE, Lewin NA, et al, eds: *Goldfrank's toxicologic emergencies,* ed 6, Stamford, CT, 1998, Appleton and Lange, pp 603-613.

Chapter 7

Organophosphate Pesticides

CHANAH DeLISLE

Organophosphates

Overview

Organophosphates (OPs) are used as pesticides, medical treatments, and chemical warfare agents. In medicine, they are currently used for the treatment of glaucoma, Alzheimer's disease, and myasthenia gravis. The most common exposure is agricultural. Over 1 million tons of pesticides are applied to U.S. crops each year. OPs inhibit acetylcholinesterase (AChE) and several other carboxylic ester hydrolases (e.g., pseudocholinesterase, chymotrypsin). Symptoms usually appear within a few hours but may immediately cause cholinergic crisis. In the case of lipid-soluble OPs, cholinergic crisis may not appear for as long as 96 hours after very mild initial symptoms. The victim can be poisoned by inhalation; by transdermal, transconjunctival, and transmucosal routes; or by injection. Inhalation is generally the most rapid route; transdermal is the slowest. OPs bind irreversibly to cholinesterase. This causes phosphorylation and deactivation of acetylcholinesterase. Acetylcholine then accumulates in the synapse, causing hyperstimulation, exhaustion, and subsequent disruption of nerve impulses.

Substances

Classification	Example	Comments
Phosphorylcholines Fluorophosphates	Echothiophate iodide Sarin	Used to treat glaucoma WMD—nerve agent
Halophosphates, cyanophosphates	Dimefox, Mipafox Tabun	Insecticide WMD—nerve agent
Dimethoxy	Malathion, parathion-methyl, dichlorvos, chlorothion, temephos	Insecticides. Malathion and parathion require "activation" within the body
Diethoxy	Diazenon, parathion, TEPP	Insecticide. Parathion is too toxic for home use.

WMD, Weapons of mass destruction.

Toxicity

Inhibition of acetylcholinesterase (AChE) is responsible for the predominant clinical effects of OP poisoning.

- Toxicity is variable depending on the agent, its affinity for enzyme inhibition, and the amount and duration of exposure.
- Chronic toxicity can occur if antidotal treatment is delayed and can lead to polyneuropathy and behavioral and personality changes.

Clinical Presentation

Cholinergic Toxidrome

See Section 3 on Mnemonics (Box 7-1).

Laboratory Evaluation

- Diagnosis is clinical.
- Electrolytes, blood urea nitrogen (BUN), creatinine to assess fluid status
- Other labs as patient's condition dictates

BOX 7-1 ▪ SIGNS AND SYMPTOMS OF ORGANOPHOSPHATE POISONING

Muscarinic effects (parasympathetic)

Bradycardia
Hypotension
Increased sweating, salivation, lacrimation, and bronchial secretions
Pulmonary edema
Nausea, vomiting, cramping, diarrhea, fecal and urinary incontinence
Wheeze, bronchoconstriction
Blurred vision, miosis (occasionally unequal)

Nicotinic effects (somatic and sympathetic)

Fasciculations, muscle twitching
Muscle weakness, cramping
Hyperglycemia, tachycardia, mydriasis, hypertension
Pallor
Paralysis, areflexia, uncoordinated respiratory efforts, respiratory failure

Central Nervous System

Emotional lability (lethargy, excitability, drowsiness)
Slurred speech, ataxia
Psychosis, delirium
Seizure*
Coma*
Death*

The final common pathway: seizure ⇒ coma ⇒ death.

- Red blood cell (RBC) cholinesterase level (EDTA tube) as baseline for future comparison
- EKG
- Chest radiograph

Treatment

- Decontaminate the victim.
  - Use nitrile or neoprene gloves; if these are not available, use double gloves.
  - Remove the victim's clothes. Use hypochlorite solution to decontaminate and then discard clothing.
  - Wash victim gently with nongermicidal soap. Rapid cleaning of the patient is more important than any specific cleaning agent.
  - Irrigate eyes with copious amounts of normal saline, lactated Ringer's solution, or tap water if eye irrigation is indicated.

- **Avoid contamination of healthcare providers**.
- **Attend to basics**: airway, breathing, circulation.
  - Continuous oximetry, cardiac monitor, establish IV access
  - Replace fluids only as needed.
  - Administer activated charcoal—1 gm/kg orally.
- Treatment may depend on degree of toxicity (see Table 7-1).

Atropine

- Noncompetitive antagonist of acetylcholine at muscarinic and CNS receptors
  - Adults: 1–2 mg IV
  - Pediatrics: 0.05 mg/kg IV
  - Double this dose every 5 min.
  - Titrate to drying of bronchial secretions.
- Alternative
  - Adults: 1 mg IV initial dose, then 2–4 mg IV q 15 min
  - Pediatrics: 0.015 mg/kg IV initial dose, then 0.015–0.05 mg/kg IV q 15 min
  - Titrate to drying of bronchial secretions.
- Extremely high doses (hundreds of milligrams) may be required.
- Drip of 2 mg/kg/hr has been reported (adult).
- Once adequately atropinized, titrate dose to maintain effect for 24 hr.
- Patient must be watched for at least 24 hr after last dose of atropine.

Table 7-1 TOXICITY AND TREATMENT OF ORGANOPHOSPHATE EXPOSURE

Degree of Toxicity	Signs and Symptoms	Treatment
Mild	Nausea, malaise, fatigue, **no diarrhea**, muscle cramping, minimal weakness	Remove from toxin until acetylcholinesterase is 7% of baseline
Moderate	SLUDGE and/or tremor, weakness, confusion, fasciculations, lethargy, anxiety, bronchorrhea	Atropine to clear bronchial secretions. 2-PAM, 1 g IV q 4–6 hr for a minimum of 24 hr or until symptoms resolve
Severe	SLUDGE, weakness, fasciculations, coma, respiratory insufficiency, paralysis, seizure, autonomic dysfunction	Atropine, benzodiazepines, 2-PAM infusion. 2-PAM for 24–48 hr until symptoms clear, longer for fat soluble or as indicated by EMG

SLUDGE, **S**alivation **L**acrimation **U**rination **D**iarrhea **G**I complaints **E**mesis.

- Tachycardia is **not** a contraindication to atropine.
- Atropine might be more helpful than endotracheal intubation and positive end expiratory pressure in the treatment of excessive secretions and respiratory distress during the acute cholinergic crisis.
- Atropine does not reactivate cholinesterase enzymes.

Pralidoxime (2-PAM)

- Reverses phosphorylation of cholinesterase and reactivates acetylcholinesterase. **Administer as soon as diagnosis is made**.
  - Adults: 1–2g IV over 15–30 min
    - May repeat in 1 hr if necessary or start a drip at 500 mg/hr.
  - Pediatrics: 25 mg/kg IV over 15–30 min, follow with continuous infusion of 10–20 mg/kg IV
  - Continue therapy until muscle weakness resolves and atropine is no longer required.
- Resolution can occur in 10–40 min or may persist for days.
- Can be administered IM or PO but to less effect.
- If necessary, wean infusion by 25% every 8 hr. Reload 1 g for breakthrough symptoms.

Seizures often respond to atropine and 2-PAM. Benzodiazepines are the next line of treatment (Table 7-2).

Special Considerations

Carbamates

The presentation of carbamate toxicity is similar to that of an organophosphate poisoning. Carbamates, however, bind reversibly to cholinesterase. Treatment with atropine is often adequate and the use of pralidoxime is controversial. Symptoms are relatively brief, resolving in hours.

Parathion

- Check serum or urine pancreatic enzymes and image patient to monitor for a painless but generally fatal pancreatitis.
- Serum hemoperfusion may be therapeutic.

Intermediate Syndrome

- Usually associated with fenthione, parathion, or malathion
- Occurs 24–96 hr after the apparent resolution of symptoms

Table 7-2 BENZODIAZEPINES DOSING FOR ADULTS AND CHILDREN

	Adult Dosing	Pediatric Dosing
Diazepam	5–10 mg IV over 3–5 min	**30 days to 5 years old**: 0.2–0.5 mg IV slowly q 2–5 min until symptoms resolve, not to exceed 5 mg
		> 5 years old: 1 mg IV q 2–5 min slowly, not to exceed 10 mg
Lorazepam	2–4 mg IV, titrate to effect	**Children:** 0.02–0.1 mg/kg IV
		Adolescents: same as adults
	Status epilepticus: 4 mg IV, may repeat in 10 min, do not exceed 8 mg	**Status epilepticus in neonates:** 0.05 mg/kg IV over 2–5 min, may repeat in 10 min
		Infants and children: 0.1 mg/kg IV over 2–5 min, not to exceed 4 mg. Second dose, 0.05 mg/kg IV at 10 min
		Adolescents: 0.7 mg/kg IV over 2–5 min, not to exceed 4 mg, may repeat in 10 min

- Sudden respiratory paralysis and neck and proximal limb muscle weakness. Grip strength is preserved.
- Hyporeflexia
- Decremental conduction on EMG with repetitive stimulation
- Not responsive to atropine or oximes
- Death due to respiratory arrest

Pediatric Considerations

- Presenting complaint is often seizure. Add organophosphate poisoning to your differential diagnosis for a child with no history of seizure who presents in status epilepticus or coma.
- Given the "leaky" nature of organophosphate poisoning, remember that children are at higher risk for dehydration. They can also become significantly hypothermic with prolonged decontamination.
- Nerve gases, such as sarin, are heavier than air and therefore more concentrated closer to the floor or at toddler height.
- Some recommend diazepam be given for exposures, even if the child is not seizing (see Table 7-2 for dosing).

Succinylcholine

If considering intubation, **remember** that succinylcholine will have a prolonged effect and the patient may be resistant to a nondepolarizing agent (vecuronium, pancuronium).

Admission Criteria

- Patients presenting with a suicide attempt
- Significant exposure requiring antidotes or intubation

Pearls and Pitfalls

- If recognized and treated rapidly, the outcome for OP-poisoned patients is good.
- Untreated, the poisoned patient will die within 24 hours.
- Unsuccessfully treated patients die within 10 days.
- When death occurs, it is usually due to respiratory failure.
- A patient should not return to work in the vicinity of the pesticides until acetylcholinesterase levels are 75% of normal.
- Significantly poisoned patients may require a **large** amount of atropine. If the patient is still wet, use generous amounts of atropine. Remember, some may require hundreds of milligrams of atropine (these would be considered good toxicity learning cases).

References and Suggested Readings

1. Aaron CK: Organophosphates and carbamates. In Ford MD, Delaney KA, Ling LJ, Erickson T et al, eds: *Clinical toxicology*, Philadelphia, 2001, WB Saunders, pp 819-828.
2. Clark RF: Insecticides: organic phosphorus compounds and carbamates. In Goldfrank LR, Flomenbaum N, Lewin N, et al, eds: *Goldfrank's toxicologic emergencies,* ed 7, New York, 2002, McGraw-Hill, pp 1346-1365.
3. Eisenstein EM, Amitai Y: Index of suspicion. Case 1. Organophosphate intoxication. *Pediatr Rev* 21:205-206, 2000.
4. Leikin JB, Thomas RG, Walter FG, et al: A review of nerve agent exposure for the critical care physician. *Crit Care Med* 30:2346-2354, 2002.
5. Nishijima DK, Wiener SW. Toxicity, organophosphate and carbamate. http://www.emedicine.com/emerg/topic346.htm. Last updated: May 11, 2006. Accessed on May 28, 2006.
6. Okumura T, Takasu N, Ishimatsu S, et al: Report on 640 victims of the Tokyo subway sarin attack, *Ann Emerg Med* 28:129-135, 1996.
7. Reigart JR, Roberts JR: Pesticides in children. *Pediatr Clin North Am* 26:377-391, 2001.
8. Sanborn MD: Identifying and managing adverse health effects: 4. Pesticides. *CMAJ* 166:1431-1436, 2002.
9. Shenoi R: Chemical warfare agents. *Clin Ped Emerg Med* 3:239-247, 2002.
10. Trujillo MH: Pharmacologic antidotes in critical care medicine: a practical guide for drug administration. *Crit Care Med* 26:377-391, 1998.

Chapter 8

Cardiovascular Drugs

BRADLEY GORDON

1. Calcium Channel Blockers

Overview

Calcium channel blockers (CCBs) work to block receptors that allow influx of Ca^{++} ions into the smooth muscle and cardiac cells. The results are decreased cardiac rate (chronotropic effect), decreased conduction through the AV node (dromotropic effect), decreased cardiac contraction (inotropic effect), and decreased smooth muscle tone of the peripheral vessels.

Substances

	Peak Effect (h) [SR*]	Bioavai- lability	Elimi- nation	$t_{1/2}$ (h)	Protein Bound
Verapamil	2.2 [5–7]	10%	Hepatic	3–7	80%–92%
Diltiazem	1.8–4.7 [6–11]	30%–60%	Hepatic	3.1–4.9	70%–80%
Nifedipine	0.5 [6]	52%–77%	Hepatic	2–5	90%–98%
Amlodipine	6–12	60%–65%	Hepatic	35–65	93%

Toxicity

- Toxicity of CCBs is variable; low-dose ingestions have caused fatalities, and high-dose ingestions have resulted in survival
  - All little as 140 mg of amlodipine caused the death of a 15-year-old girl

- Ingestion of one or two pills by a toddler has reportedly caused death
- Crushing or chewing sustained released formulations can lead to rapid onset of severe toxicity.

Clinical Presentation

See Table 8-1 for an overview of cardiovascular presentation. Other dysrhythmias include the following:

- Sinus tachycardia (specifically nifedipine)
- Atrial arrhythmias
- Junctional rhythms

Central nervous system (CNS) signs may include the development of seizures and lethargy. Patients who are asymptomatic after 6 to 8 hours post-ingestion of an immediate release product are unlikely to develop symptoms. Likewise, if a patient is without symptoms for 18 hours after ingestion of a modified release product they can be considered medically stable (the exception is verapamil, which may cause symptoms 24 hours post-ingestion).

Laboratory Evaluation

- Consider acetaminophen level (possible coingestant).
- Electrolytes, glucose, blood urea nitrogen (BUN), creatinine.
- ECG and consider chest radiograph.
- Consider salicylate level if signs of salicylism are present (see Chapter 1).

Treatment

Decontamination

- Gastric lavage in serious ingestions within 1–2 hr postingestion

Table 8-1 FREQUENCY OF SYMPTOMS ASSOCIATED WITH CCBs

Effect	Verapamil	Nifedipine	Diltiazem
Hypotension	53%	32%	38%
Depressed SA note activity	29%	14%	29%
AV block	55%	18%	29%

- Activated charcoal (AC)
  - Multidose AC considered in sustained-release preparations
- Whole bowel irrigation in sustained-release preparations

Pharmacologic Management

- Calcium ion (remember, extravasation of calcium chloride will lead to tissue necrosis)
  - Raises extracellular ionized calcium, which competitively binds calcium receptors
  - Efficacy
    - 80% of patients with hypotension responded.
    - 71% of patients with AV block responded.
    - 64% of patients with SA node suppression responded.
  - Dosing of calcium chloride (10% solution)
    - Begin with 1–3 g $CaCl_2$ IV bolus.
    - Then proceed with IV infusion at 20 to 50 mg/kg/hr of $CaCl_2$ in NS.
  - The goal for plasma calcium is 12–13 mEq/L (2–3 mEq/L ionized).
    - Check level at 30 min after start, then q 2 hr.
  - Dose range: 4.5–95.2 mEq (0.5–7 g)
  - $CaCl_2$ preferred
    - $CaCl_2$ has 3× more calcium per volume than calcium gluconate.
    - These patients may require invasive hemodynamic monitoring with a pulmonary artery catheter to optimize pharmacologic therapy.
    - $CaCl_2$ produces better plasma-ionized calcium levels.
    - 10% $CaCl_2$ has 13.6 mEq (1 g) in a 10-mL vial; calcium gluconate has 4.53 mEq in a 10-mL vial.
- Atropine
  - Blocks vagal nerve outflow, decreasing its inhibition of heart rate and cardiac output
  - 29% of patients had beneficial responses.
  - Dose range: 0.5–1 mg IV initially, dose to 3 mg total in adult
- Glucagon
  - Increases intracellular cAMP, which increases intracellular calcium concentration and as a result increases cardiac and smooth muscle contractility
  - Dosing
    - Initial dose: 3 mg (0.05 mg/kg) IV bolus
    - IV infusion: 5 mg/hr (0.07 mg/kg/hr), then titrate to

maximum of 10 mg/hr (parameter: blood pressure [BP], heart rate [HR], or both)
- Notify the pharmacy early that more glucagon may be required.
- Vasopressors
  - Dopamine at 5–20 µg/kg/min, but frequently will not sustain BP alone
  - Norepinephrine frequently added, dosed 0.5–30 µg/min IV infusion
  - Isoproterenol may be considered in refractory cases; dose range is 2–10 µg/min.
  - Phosphodiesterase inhibitors also increase cAMP levels and may be considered in refractory cases.
    - Amrinone: 0.75 mg/kg IV load over 10–15 min
      - 5–15 µg/kg/min IV infusion (titrated)
- Insulin
  - Recent evidence is quite promising.
  - No clear mechanism for the positive inotropic effect of insulin has been established, but some data point to increased calcium entry into myocytes.
  - Currently used when symptoms are refractory to other treatments, but this may change.
  - Dose: Recommend starting dose is 0.5 U/kg/hr IV infusion.
    - Usually, effects are not seen until 1 U/kg/hr.
    - Up to 10 U/kg/hr has been used.
    - Some clinicians start with 10-U IV push before infusion.
    - Monitor blood glucose q 30 min × 4 hr, then q 1 h. Supplement with dextrose at dose of 1g/kg/hr. (D10 = 10% dextrose = 10 G/100 mL.)
    - Peak effect is usually seen within 10 to 15 min (may be longer at lower doses).
  - Serum potassium will decrease. Some authors recommend "revising" reference range in these patients to 2.8–3.2 mEq/L and not supplementing until below 2.5 mEq/L. Remember, insulin drives K into the cell; there is not a total body deficit of K.

Refractory Treatments

- Invasive treatments for toxin-induced cardiogenic shock have been used, although quite infrequently.
- Intraaortic balloon counterpulsation has been implemented.
- Extracorporeal membrane oxygenation (ECMO) maybe effective until toxin has been cleared.

Special Considerations

- Extended-release and enteric-coated preparations
  - These agents may lead to delayed and prolonged toxicity. Therefore patients may require an extended period of observation, up to 24 hr postingestion. Amlodipine is especially long acting, with a half-life of up to 45 hr.
- Pediatric ingestions
  - Deaths have been reported in pediatric patients who took 1 or 2 CCB pills.
  - Aggressive therapy may be necessary in this group due to the potential for severe morbidity and mortality from seemingly small ingestions.

Admission Criteria

- Usual recommendation: Any child with any exposure should be observed for 8 hr in cases of immediate-release CCB ingestion and 24 hr in cases of sustained-release CCB ingestion.
- Most adults should be admitted to ICU for similar timeframes as in children.
- Abrupt deterioration has been reported in cases of CCB ingestion.

Pearls and Pitfalls

- Nifedipine can cause tachycardia initially.
- Extended-release products can have delayed symptoms (i.e., up to 24 hours postingestion).
- Calcium treatment is generally started too low, and initial dosing could be 2–3 g.

References and Suggested Readings

1. Boyer EW, Shannon M: Treatment of calcium channel blocker intoxication with insulin infusion, *N Engl J Med* 344:1721-1722, 2001.
2. Horowitz BZ: Calcium channel blocker toxicity, *eMedicine* 2(9), 2001.
3. Kerns W II, Kline J, Ford MD: Beta-blocker and calcium channel blocker toxicity, *Emerg Med Clin North Am* 12:365-390, 1994.
4. Pearigen PD, Benowitz NL: Poisoning due to calcium antagonists. Experience with verapamil, diltiazem and nifedipine, *Drug Safety* 6:408-430, 1991.
5. Ramoska EA, Spiller HA, Winter M, et al: A 1-year evaluation of calcium channel blocker overdoses: toxicity and treatment, *Ann Emerg Med* 22:196-200, 1993.
6. Yuan TH, Kerns WP II, Tomaszewski CA, et al: Insulin-glucose as adjunctive therapy for severe calcium channel antagonist poisoning, *J Clin Toxicol* 37:463-474, 1999.

2. β-Adrenergic Receptor Antagonists

BRADLEY GORDON

Overview

Beta receptor antagonists are used for multiple medical conditions and are therefore widely available. Although predominantly used for cardiovascular effects, they are used to treat certain anxiety reactions, essential tremors, glaucoma, migraine headaches, and thyrotoxicosis. The mechanism of effect involves the blockade of β-adrenergic receptors. Toxicity primarily affects cardiotoxicity via cardiovascular β-1 receptors. (See Table 8-2.)

Substances

Drug	Strength
Acebutolol	200 or 400 mg (capsule)
Atenolol	25, 50, or 100 mg (tablet); 5 mg/10 mL (amp)
Betaxolol	2.5 or 5 mg/mL (ophthalmic); 10 or 20 mg (tablet)
Bisprolol	5 or 10 mg (tablet)
Carteolol	2.5 or 5 mg (tablet)
Esmolol	250 mg/mL (injection)
Labetalol	100, 200, or 300 mg (tablet); 5 mg/mL (injection)
Levobunolol	0.5% (ophthalmic)
Metipranolol	0.3% (ophthalmic)
Metoprolol	50 or 100 mg (tablet); 1 mg/mL (injection)
Nadolol	20, 40, 80, 120, 160 mg (tablet)
Penbutolol	20 mg (tablet)
Pindolol	5 or 10 mg (tablets)
Propranolol	10, 20, 40, 60, 80, or 90 mg (tablet); 60, 80, 120, or 160 mg (sustained-release capsule); 1 mg/mL (injection); 80 mg/mL (oral solution)
Timolol	0.25% or 0.5% (ophthalmic); 5, 10, or 20 mg (tablet)

Adapted from MICROMEDEX(R) Healthcare Series Vol. 122 expires 12/2004.

The following agents are not available in the United States: Bupranolol, Alprenolol, Disoprolol, Tolamolol, Oxprenolol, Practolol (remember BAD TOP).

Table 8-2 PHARMACOKINETIC

	Peak (hr)	$T_{1/2}$ (hr)	Urinary Clearance
Atenolol	2–4	6–9	40%
Metoprolol	1–2	3–4	3%

▌ Toxicity

Generally, patients without heart disease are more tolerant to an overdose (OD), but there is a great deal of variability in response, even among the so-called healthy patients.

- Competitively block the β-adrenergic receptor sites.
- Depending on the drug, there is preference for β-1 (primarily in the heart) and β-2 receptors (primarily in bronchial smooth muscle and blood vessels).
  - No agent is 100% purely β-1 or β-2, and great overlap exists in OD.
- Massive ingestions of propranolol, oxprenolol, pindolol, metoprolol (somewhat), alprenolol, or acebutolol may result in "quinidine"-like or local anesthetic effect on the action potential.
- Propranolol can cause inhibition of catechol-induced glycogenolysis, which can impair the compensatory response in treated diabetics and mask the signs of hypoglycemia.
- High lipid solubility is characteristic of several β-blockers. This is important because the ability to cross the blood–brain barrier is high, and there is rapid concentration of the drug in the brain. Thus CNS toxicity occurs. Agents that are more hydrophilic are less likely to cause significant CNS toxicity (Box 8-1).
- Some β-blockers have partial agonist or intrinsic sympathomimetic activity (Box 8-2).
  - Less cardiopulmonary effect
- Chinese men have been found to have a twofold greater sensitivity to propranolol than Caucasian patients.

Box 8-1 ▪ LIPID SOLUBILITY		
Lowest Degree	**Moderate Degree**	**Highest Degree**
Nadolol	Metoprolol	Propranolol
Atenolol	Pindolol	Alprenolol
Timolol	Practolol	

Box 8-2 ▪ Partial Agonist or Intrinsic Sympathomimetic Activity	
Pindolol (greatest)	Acebutolol
Oxprenolol	Penbutolol
Alprenolol	Practolol
Carteolol	

Clinical Presentation

The prevalence of symptoms in one study was as follows:

- Bradycardia: 92%
- Hypotension: 77%
- Seizures: 58%
- EKG
  - Sinus or nodal bradycardia
  - First-degree AV block
  - QRS prolongation (slight)
  - QT prolongation

Other presentations have included hyperglycemia and lactic acidosis.

Laboratory Evaluation

- Chemistry panel, glucose
- EKG monitoring with close monitoring of vital signs

Treatment

Attend to ABCs as usual and the patient will require CNS monitoring due to development of seizures.

Decontamination

- Lavage in serious ingestion within 1–2 hr
- Multidose AC and/or whole bowel irrigation may be indicated in sustained-release preparations.

Antidotes

- Glucagon (not consistently effective and is losing favor as an antidote)

- Mechanism
  - Promotes cAMP production, which has inotropic and chronotropic effect via an increase in intracellular calcium ion concentration
  - May have an effect independent of cAMP
- Dosing
  - Initial dose: 3 mg (0.05 mg/kg) IV bolus
  - IV infusion: 5 mg/hr (0.07 mg/kg/hr), then titrate to maximum of 10 mg/hr (parameter: BP, HR, or both)
- Notify the pharmacy early that more glucagon may be required.
- Side effects
  - Nausea: Pretreat with antiemetic. Usually transient effect (i.e., minutes)
- Hypokalemia: Monitor potassium levels frequently because glucagon induces potassium shift.
- Hypoglycemia, hyperglycemia
- Generally, blood glucose rises slightly during glucagon treatment, but it is of little clinical importance in a nondiabetic patient.
- Monitor glucose in the period after discontinuing glucagon therapy because rebound hypoglycemia can occur.
- Atropine: frequently not effective as monotherapy
- Dose 0.5–1 mg IV, repeat to 3 mg maximal dose

Catecholamines

- Dopamine: Please refer to dose guidelines for calcium channel blockers.
- Isoproterenol: Please refer to dose guidelines for calcium channel blockers.

Insulin

- This therapy has shown promise in patients with calcium channel blocker toxicity and may be of benefit in β-blocker toxicity. Currently, this is only supported by animal studies, and no human use in β-blocker overdose is reported.
- Please refer to dose guidelines for calcium channel blockers and also contact your poison center for guidance.

Pacing

- May be effective in refractory cases

Special Considerations

Sotalol

- A unique β-blocker that can lead to ventricular dysrhythmias
- Considered a class III antidysrhythmic agent

Disposition

- Medical clearance can be safely made after an 8- to 10-hr observation period if there are no EKG changes and the patient remains asymptomatic with normal vital signs.

Pearls and Pitfalls

- Immediate-release preparations show signs of toxicity quickly, almost always within 6 hr.
- Sustained-release preparations must be monitored for at least 24 hr.

References and Suggested Readings

1. Kones RJ, Phillips JH: Insulin: fundamental mechanism of action and the heart, *Cardiology* 60:280-303, 1993.
2. Peterson CD, Leeder JS, Sterner S: Glucagon therapy for beta-blocker overdose, *Drug Intel* 18:394-398, 1984.
3. Roth B: Beta-blocker toxicity, *eMedicine* 2(9), 2001.
4. Weinstein RS: Recognition and management of poisoning with beta-adrenergic blocker agents, *Ann Emerg Med* 13:1123-1131, 1984.

3. Digoxin

Marny Benjamin

Overview

Causes include intentional overdose (acute overdose), chronic toxicity (due to dose error in older adults, drug interactions, or renal impairment), and plant or herbal ingestion (mostly in children under age 6 years). Cases of plant or herbal toxicity have included oleander, foxglove, yew berry, lily of the valley, dogbane,[*] Siberian ginseng, and red squill.

Digoxin's mechanism of action is to inhibit active transport of Na^+ and K^+ across cell membranes by binding the $NA + -K + -ATPase$ pump and inhibition of the Na^+ pump. Digoxin also increases the force of cardiac contraction (positive inotrope) by increasing intracellular Ca^{++}.

Kinetics

- Elimination time: 0.5–1.6 days
- Renal excretion (60%–80%) of unchanged drug, limited hepatic metabolism

Substances

CARDIAC GLYCOSIDES
Digoxin (Lanoxin)
Digitalis plant sources:
Foxglove *(Digitalis purpurea)*
Lily of the valley *(Convallaria majalis)*
Oleander *(Nerium oleander)*
Digitalis lanata
Strophanthus kombé/gratis
Hispidus seeds
Squill *(Urginea maritima, indica* bulbs)*
Dogbane *(Apocynum cannabinum)*
Digitoxin (available in Canada)

- V_d 6–7 L/kg adults, 10–16 L/kg infants
- 25% protein bound

---

[*] *Dogbane is found on the plains and foothills of the western United States, typically near streams, sandy soil, ditches, and creek beds.*

Toxicity

- **Cardiac:** Alterations in cardiac rate and rhythm may present almost any type of dysrhythmia. No particular rhythm is diagnostic, but digoxin should be suspected if increased automaticity and depressed conduction occur. The most common effect is premature ventricular contractions.
- Serum level above the normal level of 0.5–2.0 ng/mL is suspicious but not indicative of digoxin toxicity. False-positive digoxin levels refer to digoxin-like immunoreactive substances that interact with some commercially available assays used to measure digoxin levels. Patients with chronic renal insufficiency (CRI), congestive heart failure (CHF), subarachnoid hemorrhage (SAH), liver disease, acromegaly and insulin dependent diabetes mellitus (IDDM), as well as neonates, produce these substances.

Clinical Presentation

- Acute versus chronic presentation (Table 8-3)
- **Noncardiac:** anorexia, confusion, N/V, abdominal pain, HA, altered K^+ levels, visual disturbances including yellow halos (xanthopsia)
- **Degree of hyperkalemia** correlates directly with mortality.

Table 8-3 ACUTE VS. CHRONIC PRESENTATIONS OF DIGOXIN TOXICITY		
	Acute	Chronic
Typical patient	Younger without cardiac disease	Elderly with cardiac disease
Symptoms	N/V	N/V, visual, confusion, malaise, weakness
EKG	SVT w/ block and bradycardia	Ventricular dysrhythmia (bidirectional V-tach, nodal tachycardia, atrial tach w/ AV dissociation
Labs	Normal or hyperkalemia	Normal or hypokalemia (depends on use of loop diuretics)
Digoxin level	High	High normal or slightly elevated

Laboratory Evaluation

- 12-lead EKG and continuous cardiac monitoring
- Check electrolytes and digoxin level.

Treatment

- **Stop digoxin**.
- Activated charcoal (consider MDAC)
- Consider contacting poison center or toxicologist to aid in management.
- Electrolyte management
  - Hyperkalemia ≥ 5.0 digoxin-Fab therapy. If digoxin-specific Fab fragments are not available, aggressively treat hyperkalemia with insulin/glucose and HCO_3.
  - Hypokalemic: IV KCl until low normal
  - Hypomagnesemia: replete with IV $MgSO_4$
  - Hypocalcemia: Avoid replacement because intracellular calcium is often very high.
- Dysrhythmia management
  - Supraventricular tachydysrhythmias: β-blockers with/without digoxin-specific Fab fragments
  - Supraventricular bradydysrhythmias: atropine with/without digoxin-specific Fab fragments
  - High-degree AV block: digoxin-specific Fab fragments
  - V tach/fib: defibrillation, digoxin-specific Fab fragments, lidocaine/amiodarone, phenytoin, $MgSO_4$
  - **Avoid isoproterenol and calcium (risk of cardiac tetany).**

Digoxin-Specific Antibody Fragments (Fab, Digibind, DigiFab)

- Safe (although can exacerbate CHF if CHF patients are given too much)
- Onset 19–88 min
- Digoxin levels cannot be correlated clinically after Digibind administration because most assays measure bound and unbound digoxin.
- Recurrent toxicity can occur in patients with renal failure up to 10 days after administration of Digibind. **Hemodialysis does not enhance its elimination.**
- Indications and dosing
  - Ventricular dysrhythmias
  - Progressive brady-dysrhythmias that are unresponsive to atropine. High grade AV block is a serious prognostic factor.

- Potassium concentration ≥5.5 mEq/L in setting of suspected acute digoxin toxicity
- Rapidly progressive cardiac dysrhythmias with hemodynamic compromise or a rising potassium concentration
- Serum digoxin concentration ≥15 ng/mL at any time, or ≥10 ng/mL at steady state
- Ingestion of ≥10 mg in an adult or ≥4 mg in a child
- Unknown ingestion with characteristics suggestive of digoxin, calcium channel blocker, or β-blocker overdose
- Dose: Administer digoxin immune Fab (DigiFab, Protherics, Nashville, TN) by IV infusion over 30 min using an inline 0.22-μm membrane filter. If cardiac arrest is imminent, give quickly as a bolus injection.
  - Calculations:
    - **Based on amount ingested acutely:** Number of vials = (mg ingested × 0.8) ÷ 0.5
    - **Based on digoxin level:** No. of vials = serum digoxin level (ng/mL) × V_d × patient weight (kg) ÷ 1000 × 0.5 mg/vial
    - **Estimated:** number of vials = serum dig level (ng/mL) × patient weight (kg) ÷ 100
  - Empiric: Acute ingestion
    - Adult: 10–20 vials
    - Child: 10–20 vials
  - Chronic ingestion
    - Adult: 3–6 vials
    - Child: 1/4–1/2 vial
  - Consider half-dose in chronic toxicity patients, especially those with CHF.

Special Considerations

- Chronic digoxin toxicity
  - See "Treatment."
- Plant toxicity
  - Plants containing digitalis glycosides may be treated with digoxin-immune Fab.

Admission Criteria

- Admit to ICU or CCU if any signs of toxicity, dysrhythmia, or if patient received Digibind or DigiFab.
- Patients with accidental exposures with no signs of toxicity after 12 hours can be discharged and can be discharged home.

Pearls and Pitfalls

- Certain plants can cause toxicity similar to digoxin overdose.
- Consider coingestions in acute overdose cases.
- Patients with digoxin toxicity are frequently diagnosed as having dementia, depression, dehydration, acute confusional state, or psychosis.
- Certain medical conditions may cause release of digoxin-like immune substances, leading to misdoses of digoxin toxicity and delayed medical diagnosis.
- In chronic toxicity, the number of vials roughly equals the digoxin level.

References and Suggested Readings

1. Lewin NA: Cardiac glycosides. In Goldfrank LR, Flomenbaum N, Lewin N, et al, eds: *Goldfrank's toxicologic emergencies,* ed 6. New York, 1998, McGraw-Hill.
2. Howland MA: Digoxin-specific antibody fragments (Fab).
3. Dribben WH, Kirk MA: Digitalis glycosides. In Tintinalli JE, Kelen GD, Stapczynski JS, eds: *Emergency medicine: a comprehensive study guide,* ed 5. New York, 2000, McGraw-Hill.

Chapter 9

Drugs of Abuse

Carson R. Harris

1. Cocaine

Overview

Cocaine has a long history of use and abuse, dating to the sixth century. It is a natural product, but not a "nutritional supplement," from the leaves of the coca plant. Cocaine is used for medical and nonmedical purposes. Most of the illicit cocaine in the United States comes from South America. Cocaine causes sympathomimetic toxidrome (see "Toxidrome"), with effects of tachycardia, hyperthermia, hypertension, seizures, diaphoresis, and mydriasis. Nearly every organ system of the body is affected. Cocaine's mechanisms of actions are sympathomimetic and atherogenic. Cocaine can be smoked (e.g., crack, freebase), injected, or snorted (e.g., cocaine hydrochloride). Some of its kinetics are listed in Table 9-1.

Toxicity

- The LD50 of cocaine has been reported as being 2 g. However, seasoned addicts may tolerate up to 10 g/day without serious acute toxicity.
- Alcohol and cocaine form **cocaethylene**, which may be more toxic to the organs (brain and heart) than cocaine alone. (The literature is not consistent.)

Table 9-1 COCAINE KINETICS			
	Onset	**Peak**	**Duration**
IV, smoked	15–60 sec	5–10 min	20 min
Nasal	15–20 min	15–60 min	1.5 hr

- More euphorigenic and responsible for the intense effect of cocaine
- Most likely responsible for prolonging the effect of cocaine

Substances

- Description
  - White powder, crystal, paste
  - Rock or crack is off-white to yellowish in color.
- Cocaine paste is cocaine sulfate (a.k.a. bazooka, pasta, basuco) and can be sold for abuse or further developed into cocaine hydrochloride.
- Speedball is injected heroin and cocaine; modified speedball is injected heroin and smoked crack.
- Can be adulterated with just about anything, such as sugars, talc, lidocaine, Dilantin, and strychnine as well as other abused drugs.

- Cocaine goes to all areas of the brain, but it binds to sites in some very specific areas: the ventral tegmental area (VTA), the nucleus accumbens, and the caudate nucleus (the reward areas in the brain).
- The binding in the caudate nucleus can explain other effects such as increased stereotypic (or repetitive) behaviors (pacing, nail-biting, scratching, etc.). (You may wish to review your neuropathology notes from medical school.)
- See Figure 9-1.

Clinical Presentation

- **General**: agitated, may be disoriented
- **Vital signs**: hypertensive, tachycardia, tachypnea, hyperthermia
- **Cardiovascular**: chest pain, myocardial infarction (MI), myocarditis, angina, hypertension, sinus tachycardia, V-tach, V-fib, aortic dissection
- **Pulmonary**: chest pain, pneumothorax, pneumomediastinum, hemoptysis, crack lung (bilateral infiltrates, eosinophilia, etc.), pulmonary edema

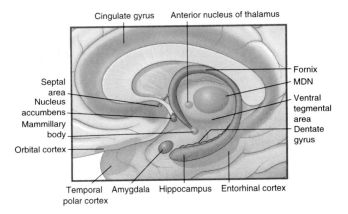

Figure 9-1 ■ Structures of the brain playing an important role in addiction and pleasure. Drug-induced release of dopamine at the ventral tegmental area (VTA) leads to a cascade of events in the "pleasure circuit." From Fitzgerald MJT, Folan-Curran J: *Clinical neuroanatomy and related neuroscience,* 4th ed. Philadelphia, 2002, WB Saunders, p 277.

- **Neurologic**: seizure, agitation, tremor, myoclonic jerking, choreoathetoid movements, cerebrovascular accident (CVA) (bleeding or ischemic)
- **Gastrointestinal**: vomiting, abdominal pain (especially in stuffers and packers), bowel ischemia or infarct (if suspected, consult surgeon and toxicologist **early**)
- **Genitourinary**: renal infarction, acute tubular necrosis (ATN), acute renal failure (ARF)
- **Pupils**: dilated
- **Psychiatric**: agitated, anxiety
- **Other concerns**
  - Rhabdomyolysis
  - **Cocaine washout syndrome**: lethargic, difficult to arouse, hypotensive, bradycardia
    - Seen in patients who binge for several days, depleting their catecholamines. Syndrome may be precipitated by giving benzodiazepines.
- **EKG**: sinus tach, V-tach, wide QRS, ST-T wave changes (elevation, inversion)

■ Laboratory Evaluation

- CBC, electrolytes, blood urea nitrogen (BUN)/creatinine, glucose
- Troponin
- Urine assay (UA), urine toxicology screen (doctors order this, but results rarely change management)
- Creatine kinase (CK) to R/O rhabdomyolysis. The urine color may be a clue to presence of myoglobin.
- EKG and monitor rhythm if patient has chest pain, shortness of breath (SOB), or abnormal rhythm
- Chest radiograph, abdominal films depending on presentation

■ Treatment

- For most ED presentations (chest pain, anxiety, supraventricular tachycardia), giving oxygen and benzodiazepines will suffice.
- Diazepam 5–10 mg IV or lorazepam 1–2 mg IV, titrate to effect
- Cardiovert unstable supraventricular tachycardia. May try diltiazem 20 mg IV or verapamil 5–10 mg IV if patient is hemodynamically stable
- Ventricular dysrhythmias
  - Sodium bicarbonate 1–2 mEq/kg IV; lidocaine 1.5 mg/kg IV, then infusion of 2–4 mg/min if initial bolus is successful
  - Defibrillate if hemodynamically unstable
- Hypertension
  - Phentolamine 1 mg IV; repeat in 5 min
  - Nitroglycerin infusion
- Acute coronary syndrome
  - O_2, acetylsalicylic acid (ASA) 325 mg, benzodiazepines, nitroglycerin 0.4 mg SL × 3 doses followed by nitroglycerin infusion
  - Morphine 2 mg IV q 5 min, titrate to pain relief. Monitor pressure, level of consciousness, and respiratory rate.
  - Phentolamine 1 mg IV, repeat in 5 min
  - Unfractionated heparin or low molecular weight heparin (LMWH)
  - Fibrinolytics (options: know what your institution uses and your cardiologist prefers)
  - PCI with glycoprotein IIb/IIIa inhibitors
- Pulmonary edema
  - Furosemide 20–40 mg IV
  - Nitroglycerin infusion titrated to BP

- Morphine 2 mg q 5 min titrated to pain relief or respiratory status
- Hyperthermia
  - Benzodiazepines, cooling techniques
  - Continuously monitor temperature (bladder thermistor catheter)
- Seizures
  - Benzodiazepines
  - Phenobarbital 25–50 mg/min
- **Controversial treatments**
  - β-blockers: leads to unopposed α-adrenergic effects (exacerbation of tachycardia and hypertension)
  - Labetalol: remember that it is an α- and β-adrenergic blocker, but it has more β than α (7:1 for IV doses). Patient may develop worsening of hypertension and tachycardia.
  - Calcium channel blockers: animal studies not very promising

Special Considerations

Packers and Stuffers

- **Body packers**: Carefully wrap cocaine and ingest the packets to transport across borders.
  - The best evidence available suggests that asymptomatic cocaine body packers can be managed conservatively until they have completely passed their packets. Close clinical observation in the meantime allows for the early detection of developing complications that may require emergency surgery.
  - Whole bowel irrigation with polyethylene glycol: Electrolyte solution (PEG-ES) such as GoLYTELY (Braintree Laboratories, Inc. Braintree, MA) has been advocated (see below).
- **Body stuffers**: Hastily wrap drug and stuff it down the throat (swallow) or into the anus or vagina to avoid being arrested with the goods.
  - If the patient is asymptomatic, use conservative management with activated charcoal with sorbitol. Some have advocated whole bowel irrigation, using (GoLYTELY) given in large quantities, to increase transit time through the gut.
  - Adults receive 1.5–2 L/hr via NG tube (it is a rare patient who sits still to drink the solution at the effective rate of 400–500 mL q 15 min).

Cocaine Washout Syndrome

- Occurs when drug use is halted (medical illness, jail, insolvency)
- Most likely a lack of CNS neurotransmitters (e.g., norepinephrine, serotonin, dopamine)
- Incidence unknown, likely quite common
- There are few data in the medical literature, but street savvy is quite knowledgeable on this topic.
- Precipitated in ED with minimal benzodiazepine administration
- Possible clinical findings
  - Vital signs normal, usually not hypotensive nor bradycardic to the point of requiring treatment
  - Signs of cocaine toxicity absent
  - Patients appear in a deep-sleep state
  - Unresponsiveness may be quite impressive
- Treatment
  - Supportive only; protect airway and vital signs
  - Stimulants not warranted
  - Course: Patients wake up slowly over 12–24 hr

Pregnancy and Cocaine

- In some states, women can be prosecuted for prenatal child abuse if they use cocaine during pregnancy.
- Involve social services and chemical dependency counselors.

Admission Criteria

- Altered mental status or seizure
- Significant hypertension or tachycardia
- Ventricular dysrhythmias
- Chest pain with positive cardiac markers; otherwise, treat and observe for 12 hr
- Pneumothorax or pneumomediastinum
- Symptomatic body stuffer or body packer
- Hyperthermia

Pearls and Pitfalls

- Benzodiazepines, benzodiazepines, benzodiazepines
- Antipyretics are not effective for hyperpyrexia due to cocaine.
- Think phentolamine for hypertension or recalcitrant ischemic chest pain.
- Severe rhabdomyolysis, leading to renal failure, can occur.

- Cocaine abuse can affect nearly every organ system of the body.
- Occasionally, burn marks or hyperkeratotic areas on the distal volar thumb(s) are an indication of crack pipe use.

References and Suggested Readings

1. Harris CR: Cocaine. In Harris CR, ed: *Emergency management of selected drugs of abuse,* Dallas, 2000, American College of Emergency Physicians.
2. Hollander JE: Management of cocaine associated myocardial ischemia, *N Engl J Med* 333:1267, 1995.
3. Hollander JE, Hoffman RS: Cocaine. In Ford MD, Delaney KA, Ling LJ, Erickson T, eds: *Clinical toxicology,* Philadelphia, 2001, Saunders.
4. Kosten TR, O'Connor PG: Management of drug and alcohol withdrawal, *N Engl J Med* 348:1786, 2003.
5. Wilson LD, Jeromin J, Garvey L, et al: Cocaine, ethanol, and cocaethylene cardiotoxicity in an animal model of cocaine and ethanol abuse, *Acad Emerg Med* 8:211, 2001.

2. Amphetamine and Methamphetamine

CHANAH DELISLE

Overview

Amphetamine and methamphetamine are phenethylamines. As central and peripheral adrenergic receptor agonists, they cause release of catecholamines and block reuptake of dopamine, norepinephrine, and serotonin. Amphetamine and methamphetamine are lipophilic, have a half-life of 8–30 hr, and undergo hepatic metabolism with a pH-dependent renal excretion. They may be ingested PO, IV, or IN. Chronic use leads to vasculitis, cardiomyopathy, and pulmonary hypertension.

Although commonly abused "street drugs," amphetamine and methamphetamine are available in prescription form and are used therapeutically for attention-deficit hyperactivity disorder, narcolepsy, and as an anorexic agent for weight loss.

Methamphetamine is easily and inexpensively produced from readily available precursors. Its popularity is increasing. The final product brings a good price on the street. Laboratories are simple and are often created in homes or garages and thus can be quickly dismantled. Inhaled methamphetamine is replacing cocaine as the drug of choice in some geographic areas. It delivers an equally intense and longer-lasting high.

AMPHETAMINE

Substances

Prescription Names for Amphetamines

Amphetamine
Dexfenfluramine
Dextroamphetamine
Fenfluramine
Methamphetamine
Methylphenidate
Pemoline
Phendimetrazine
Phentermine

Street Names for Amphetamines

Bennies
Black beauties
Crosses
Dexies
Hearts
Mollies
Purple hearts
Speed
Uppers
Whiz

Toxicity

- Ingestions in the low range of 1.3 mg/kg of amphetamine have caused death.
- Methylphenidate
  - 5 mg/kg ingestion has caused fatalities.
  - IN abuse has lead to a fatality.

- Less than 1 mg/kg ingestion of methylphenidate is reported as nontoxic in pediatric patients.
- As always, clinical presentation is more important than trying to calculate or estimate the ingested dose.

Clinical Presentation

- Patient may complain of simple headache, nausea, and/or insomnia.
- Remember that tachycardia with psychosis can imply not only amphetamine toxicity, but also an overdose of an acetaminophen/diphenhydramine preparation.
- See Box 9-1.

BOX 9-1 ▪ CLINICAL PRESENTATION OF AMPHETAMINE TOXICITY

Cardiovascular

Palpitations, tachycardia
Hypertension, hypertensive encephalopathy
Chest pain
Dysrhythmias
Myocardial ischemia; vasospasm

Neurologic

Acute psychosis, delusions, paranoia (may last for days)
Seizure
Intracranial hemorrhage, vasospasm
Hyperpyrexia
Euphoria, anxiety, life-threatening agitation
Hyperreflexia
Compulsive, repetitive behaviors (e.g., cleaning house, picking teeth)
Bruxism
Anorexia
Increased alertness, concentration; decreased fatigue

Sympathetic

Mydriasis
Diaphoresis
Nausea
Tremor
Tachypnea

Other

Rhabdomyolysis
Ischemic colitis
Pulmonary edema
Muscle rigidity
Piloerection
Urinary retention

- Other complications of amphetamine use are presented in Box 9-2.
- Acute ingestion of a massive overdose will cause initial stimulation followed by sudden CNS depression. **Death can occur in a few minutes.**

Laboratory Evaluation

- Electrolytes, arterial blood gases (ABG) (to evaluate for acidosis), CK, UA (look for "large blood, RBC 0"), rhabdomyolysis, and acetaminophen level
- 12-lead EKG if patient complains of chest pain or if co-ingestion is a concern
  - Look for ST depression or elevation to rule out myocardial ischemia or infarction in a patient with chest pain.
  - Look for clues to possible coingestions, such as the widened QRS seen in tricyclic antidepressant toxicity.
  - Head CT if altered mental status or severe headache.
  - Especially if patient complains of headache, has had a seizure, or has any neurologic abnormality.
- Chest radiograph
- Other testing dependent on presentation

Treatment

- Address the basics: airway, breathing, circulation, disability, SNOT (sugar, Narcan, oxygen, thiamine).

BOX 9-2 ▪ OTHER COMPLICATIONS OF CHRONIC AMPHETAMINE USE

Necrotizing vasculitis

Progressive necrotizing arteritis resulting in renal failure
Pancreatitis, cerebral infarction, hemorrhage

Cardiomyopathy

Heart failure, dysrhythmias, ischemia

IV drug use and potential sequelae

HIV infection, AIDS, hepatitis, endocarditis, pulmonary and soft tissue abscess, osteomyelitis

Amphetamine-induced psychosis

Can last for a few days before returning to normal; includes auditory and visual hallucinations, significant paranoia

- Take vital signs, including rectal temperature. Hyperpyrexia must be addressed immediately.

Seizures

- Benzodiazepines, barbiturates
    - **Valium** 0.2–0.4 mg/kg IV, reasonable adult dose 2.5–10 mg IV
    - **Ativan** 0.05–0.1 mg/kg IV, reasonable adult dose 2–4 mg IV/IM
    - **Phenobarbital** 15–20 mg/kg IV
    - Will rapidly control agitation. Control of the agitation will help control blood pressure, hyperthermia, and worsening or pending rhabdomyolysis.
    - Titrate to effect (high therapeutic index). Monitor airway.
    - For refractory seizures, consider **propofol,** 2.5 mg/kg followed by 0.2 mg/kg/min drip.

Hypertension

- **Nitroprusside:** start at 0.3 µg/kg/min, titrate to effect
- **Phentolamine** 5 mg IV
- Agitation control will often control hypertension.

Rhabdomyolysis

- IV fluids to maintain urine output of 1–2 mL/kg/min
- Consider buffered IV fluids, easily prepared by withdrawing 150 mL from 1 L of D_5W, then adding 3 amps $NaHCO_3$

See Table 9-2.

Table 9-2 TREATMENT SUMMARY OF AMPHETAMINE TOXICITY

Agitation	Benzodiazepines
Seizures	Benzodiazepines
	Barbiturates
Hyperthermia	Control agitation
	External cooling with mist and fans
Hypertension	Control agitation
	Vasodilator (nitroprusside)
	α-antagonist (phentolamine)
	Avoid β-blockers (unopposed α effects)
Psychosis	Benzodiazepines
	Consider neuroleptics if normal vital signs
Rhabdomyolysis	Control agitation
	External cooling
	IV fluids to maintain urine output of 1–2 mL/kg/min

■ Special Considerations

Packers and Stuffers

- **Body packers:** carefully wrap the drugs and ingest the wrapped packets to transport across borders.
- Asymptomatic amphetamine body packers probably can be managed conservatively until they have completely passed their packets. In the meantime, close clinical observation allows for the early detection of developing complications that may require emergency surgery.
- Whole bowel irrigation with polyethylene glycol. Electrolyte solution (PEG-ES) such as GoLYTELY has been advocated (see below).
- **Body stuffers:** hastily wrap drug and stuff it down the throat (swallow) or into the anus or vagina to avoid being arrested with the goods (or the bads, or the ugly).
- If the patient is asymptomatic, use conservative management with activated charcoal with sorbitol. Some have advocated whole bowel irrigation, using GoLYTELY in large quantities, to increase transit time through the gut.
- Adults receive 1.5–2 L/hr via NG tube.

Pregnancy

- Amphetamine intoxication may present as eclampsia.

■ METHAMPHETAMINES

■ Substances

Street Names for Methamphetamine*

Chalk, crank
Crystal, crystal meth
Cristy
Glass, go
Ice
Meth
Zip

Also refer to the Appendix.

Toxicity

Abusers who use heavily will consume 15–1000 times the recommended therapeutic dose.

Clinical Presentation

The clinical presentation is similar to amphetamine.
- Acute ingestion, smoking, or injection results in initial hypertension, hyperpyrexia, and hyperactivity. In a series of 127 cases, the frequency of symptoms of patients presenting to the ED included the following (see also Table 9-3):
  - HEENT
    - Dilated, slowly reactive or nonreactive pupils
    - Decreased corneal reflex
  - Cardiovascular
    - Peripheral effects
    - Atrial and ventricular arrhythmias
    - Systolic and diastolic hypertension (may be postural)
    - Palpitations and tachycardia
    - Reflex bradycardia may also occur.
    - Cardiac output is increased.
    - Myocardial ischemia and infarction, angina, and peripheral vasospasm

Table 9-3 CLINICAL EFFECTS OF CNS STIMULANT DRUGS	
Clinical Presentation	**Frequency (%)**
Hypertension	33
Agitation	22
Coma	10
Chest pain	9
Hallucinations	7
Confusion	6
Delusions	5
Weakness and lethargy	5
Headache	4
Abdominal pain	4
Palpitations	3
Seizures	3
Paresthesia	2

- Acute cardiomyopathy after IV abuse
- Respiratory
  - Tachypnea and noncardiogenic pulmonary edema after IV abuse
- Neurologic
  - Altered mental status is the most common manifestation of acute intoxication.
  - Agitation, confusion, delirium, hallucinations, dizziness, dyskinesias, hyperactivity, muscle fasciculations and rigidity, rigors, tics, and tremors
  - Seizures and coma
  - Cerebral vasculitis has been described.
  - Hemorrhagic, vasospastic, or ischemic strokes
  - Choreiform movements have occurred after acute and chronic intoxication.
- Gastrointestinal
  - Nausea, vomiting, and diarrhea
  - Abdominal cramps are common.
  - Hematemesis has occurred after IV abuse.
- Genitourinary
  - Renal failure may occur secondary to dehydration or rhabdomyolysis in overdose.
  - Polyuria, dysuria, hesitancy, and acute urinary retention
  - Hyperthermia may result due to increased metabolic and muscular activity.
- Psychiatric
  - Visual hallucinations, illusions, delusion of reference, and delusional perception in 25%–49% of patients
  - Active psychosis can last from 10 days (64% of abusers) to 6 months (10% of abusers).
- Dermatologic
  - Multiple skin excoriations caused by the user picking at his or her skin due to formication, a belief that one's skin is infested with bugs.
    - Cellulitis and skin abscesses

▎ Laboratory Evaluation

- Similar to amphetamine toxicity
- Beware of the cross-reactors on urine toxicology screens.
  - Cross-reactivity depends on the assay used by your toxicology lab, concentration in the body, and limits of the assay. Always confirm rapid toxicology screens with the most sensitive method of drug testing, GC-MS (gas chromatography–mass spectrometry).
- Urine detectability is typically 2–4 days.

Possible Cross-Reactors	
Ephedrine	MDMA (Ecstasy)
Phentermine	Procainamide
Vicks Nasal Spray (L-methamphetamine)	Ranitidine
Isoxsuprine (Vasodilan)	Selegiline

▊ Treatment

See "Amphetamines."

▊ Admission Criteria

See "Amphetamines."

Pearls and Pitfalls

- All that is tachycardic and psychotic is not amphetamine induced. The active ingredient in OTC sleep preparations is often diphenhydramine with acetaminophen.
- Get an acetaminophen level. This is also worth considering when medically clearing a psychiatric patient.
- CORE temperature. Consider rectal temperature or thermistor Foley.
- Although urinary acidification decreases half-life and increases elimination, it does not lessen the toxicity of amphetamines and would worsen renal complications of rhabdomyolysis.
- Neuroleptics may cause acute dystonia and cardiac dysrhythmias, lower seizure threshold, and alter temperature regulation. Rely on benzodiazepines for acute psychosis associated with amphetamine/methamphetamine intoxication.
- If paralysis is required to control temperature and seizures have been an issue, continuous EEG monitoring is necessary.
- Selegiline (Eldepryl), used for Parkinson's disease, is specifically metabolized to levoamphetamine and levomethamphetamine. Concentrations of L-methamphetamine in serum after therapeutic dosing (10 mg/day) with selegiline were 9–15 ng/mL. Urine concentrations were not specified, so it is unclear whether sufficient amounts are excreted to reach the cutoff level for drug abuse screening. The L-methamphetamine generated from this

drug would be expected to produce the same difficulty with laboratory confirmation as with the Vicks inhaler.
• COOL is good. (But we've all known that since seventh grade.)

References and Suggested Readings

1. Amphetamines and designer drugs. In Ellenhorn MJ, Schonwald S, Ordog G, eds: *Medical toxicology: diagnosis and treatment of human poisoning,* Baltimore, 1997, Williams and Wilkins.

2. Colucciello SA, Tomaszewski C: Substance abuse. In Rosen P, Barkin R, Danzl D, et al: *Emergency medicine concepts and clinical practice,* 4th ed. St. Louis, 1998, Mosby.

3. Derlet RW, Rice P, Horowitz BZ, Lord RV: Amphetamine toxicity: experience with 127 cases, *J Emerg Med* 7:157, 1989.

4. Heinonen EH, Rinne UK: Selegiline in the treatment of parkinson's disease, *Acta Neurol Scand Suppl* 126:103, 1989.

5. Chiang WK: Amphetamines. In Goldfrank LR, Flomenbaum NE, Lewin NA, et al, eds: *Toxicologic emergencies,* 6th ed. Stamford, CT, 1998, Appleton & Lange.

6. MacKenzie RG: Methamphetamine, *Pediatr Rev* 18:305, 1997.

7. Methamphetamine. Poisindex Management. MICROMEDEX Healthcare Series, vol 122, expired Dec 2004.

8. Zeleznikar R: Amphetamines and methamphetamine. In Harris CR, ed: *Emergency management for selected dugs of abuse,* Dallas, 2000, American College of Emergency Physicians.

3. MDMA (Ecstasy)

DAVID CHEESEBROW

Overview

MDMA is also known as 3,4-methylenedioxymethamphetamine. The goal of the user is to increase endurance of an activity such as dancing or obtain subjective pleasure such as empathy, openness, caring, euphoria, disinhibition, and increased sensuality and decrease feelings of fear, defensiveness, aggression, separation from others, and obsessiveness. MDMA is seen as a "safe" drug, and pills may have been "tested" as safe with only MDMA present. Its actions are similar to methamphetamine and mescaline. It is a selective serotonergic neurotoxin that causes massive release of serotonin and inhibits its uptake. Its route is usually oral ingestion of a white, yellow, or beige pill, often with motif symbols on the pills. It is also taken via injection or in the powder form inserted into the rectum.

Each tablet is 50–100 mg of MDMA but can range from 50–300 mg. Many pills range from 80–120 mg. Effective doses are 1–2 mg/kg. The onset is usually 30–60 minutes (referred to as "the launch"), and duration is 3–4 hours. Mood shifts can occur for several days, from elevation to depression.

Substances

Common street names include: ecstasy, XTC, Adam, E, X, "hug drug," Bean, Roll, M & M, and others (see the Appendix "Street Names for Drugs of Abuse")	Related drugs: 2,5 dimethoxy-4-methylphenyliso-propylamine (DOM, "Serenity, Tranquility, Peace" [STP])
Teens and young adults using MDMA may refer to their use as "X-ing," "rolling," "tripping," or "wigging."	Methoxyamphetamine Methylenedioxyamphetamine (MDA) Dimethoxyamphetamine (DMA) Methylenedioxy-ethylamphetamine (MDEA, "Eve," MDE) Trimethoxyamphetamine (TMA) Paramethoxyamphetamine (PMA)

Toxicity

- **CYP2D6:** An enzyme that is not found in a small percentage of the population. Patients lacking this enzyme may not be able to metabolize ecstasy.
- Severe hyperthermia reported at doses of 4–5 mg/kg. Tolerance occurs quickly, with a need to increase dosage.

Clinical Presentation

- History
  - History of a party, rave, or ingestion of ecstasy and other drugs but often not alcohol. Users are often under 21 years of age.
  - A *rave* is an all-night dance featuring techno music with a heavy beat, usually played by DJs. The term was originally used by Caribbean people living in London to describe a party.

- Patients often present to the ED late at night or early morning.
- Patients often wear a neon-colored necklace or sticks and a pacifier and carry "smart drinks," which are blends of fruit drink with amino acids.
- Present to the ED because of an adverse reaction or ingestion of other drugs. The other drugs can be but are not limited to alcohol, marijuana, ketamine, gamma-hydroxybutyrate (GHB), heroin, cocainem, or ephedrine.
- Remember that polysubstance abuse is the rule rather than the exception, so the presentation may be confusing.
- The three major signs of toxicity are **tachycardia, hypertension,** and **hyperthermia.**
- See Box 9-3.

Laboratory Evaluation

- A bedside blood glucose if patients presents in an altered mental state. Other blood work includes CBC, electrolyte studies, LFTs, coagulation studies, UA and urine toxicologic screen, ethanol, ketones, and serum osmolarity.
- EKG and chest radiograph in cases of respiratory distress
- Head CT for those with seizures or prolonged mental status changes
- Pregnancy test (in females). MDMA crosses the placenta.

Treatment

- ABCs including IV access, cardiac and oxygen saturation monitoring, blood pressure and core temperature monitoring
- If patient is interactive, provide reassurance, avoid restraints, and have a calm, quiet environment. If patient is severely disruptive or a physical danger to self or others, then sedation and restraint may be necessary.
- See Table 9-4.

Special Considerations

- Patients who are HIV positive and taking protease inhibitors have an inability to metabolize MDMA due to alterations in the P-450 systems.

BOX 9-3 ▪ PHYSICAL FINDINGS OF MDMA TOXICITY

Vital Signs

Tachycardia with dysrhythmias such as PVCs, SVT, VT, or VF
Tachypnea
Hypertensive
Hyperthermia

CNS

Altered level of consciousness from hyper-alert state to lethargy
Often in constant motion
Easily agitated with anxiety and paranoia
Headache
Blurred vision, "seeing halos"

EENT

Pupils may be small with nystagmus.
Bruxism (teeth grinding)
Dry mouth
Trismus with jaw clenching

Pulmonary

Respiratory distress
Respiratory failure
Noncardiogenic pulmonary edema

Cardiovascular

Tachycardia, palpations, chest pain and syncope

Gastrointestinal

Nausea, vomiting
Anorexia
Abdominal pain

Genitourinary

Urinary retention

Skin

Diaphoretic
Piloerection

- Patient taking MAO inhibitors can have hypertensive crisis, intracranial hemorrhage, and severe hyperthermia. This is due to excessive serotonin and norepinephrine release.
- Priapism may be due to combination of ecstasy and Viagra, known as "trail mix" in some areas of the country; also used at sextasy parties.

Table 9-4 MANAGEMENT OF MDMA TOXICITY

Condition/ Toxic Effect	Treatment	Notes
Airway	Intubation is necessary to protect airway or if respiratory distress is present.	
Decontamination	Activated charcoal PO/NG	Gastric lavage is only indicated if patient presents early after ingestion (within 1 hr) and a potentially lethal amount of ecstasy or coingestant is involved.
Hyperthermia	Use of cooling and a fan, ice packs to groin and axilla, iced gastric lavage, control shivering with a benzodiazepine	Aggressive treatment required if core temperature is over 102° F
Hypertension	Benzodiazepines	
Serotonin syndrome	(See Chapter 3, "Antidepressants")	
Rhabdomyolysis	Generous IV fluids and alkalinization of urine with sodium bicarbonate	
Disseminated intravascular coagulation (DIC)	Anticoagulant therapy, replace blood products as indicated, consider Cryoprecipitate and Antithrombin III concentrate	
Hepatotoxicity	Supportive care	Consultation with hepatologist/GI specialist
Acute renal failure	Monitor output, reassess	Consultation with renal specialist
Hyponatremia	Correct sodium. Begin fluid restriction. In severe cases, 3% saline and furosemide may be indicated. Limit to a rate of 0.5–1 mEq/L/hr. Look for a high urine osmolarity, low serum osmolarity, and hyponatremia. Signs of cerebral edema, seizures, and coma	Due to increased water intake, excessive sweating, and release of vasopressin leading to inappropriate antidiuretic syndrome (SIADH)
Neurologic effects (subarachnoid hemorrhage, cerebral infarction, or parenchymal bleed)	Supportive care	Look for these in patients with altered mental status, Thoroughly check for history of congenital AV malformations or cerebral angiomas.

Admission Criteria

- Admit all patients with serious symptoms of toxicity (i.e., seizure or altered mental status in the ED).
- Hyperthermia, electrolyte abnormality, sustained abnormal VS
- Discharge those without serious signs and symptoms who improve in the ED after 6 hr of observation. (This is an arbitrary number. There are no studies to support the timing, but the effects of ecstasy typically last 3–5 hr.)
- **The patient must be accompanied home by a responsible adult. (DO NOT send the patient back to the party!)**
- Social service evaluation

Pearls and Pitfalls

- All pills sold as "ecstasy" are **not** ecstasy and could be more toxic.
- The typical dose is 75–150 mg, but some pills are sold as a "double-stack" and contain twice as much ecstasy.
- Altered mental status and seizures may be due to hyponatremia, CNS bleed, or edema.
- Ecstasy can cause serotonin syndrome. Remember, this is diagnosis of exclusion, and other "badness" must be ruled out.
- Priapism etiology may be due to ecstasy and sildenafil (Viagra).

References and Suggested Readings

1. Baggott MJ: Preventing problems in Ecstasy users: reduce use to reduce harm, *J Psychoactive Drug* 34:145, 2002.
2. Green AR, Mechan AO, Elliott JM, et al: The pharmacology and clinical pharmacology of 3,4-methylenedioxymethamphetamine (MDMA, "ecstasy"), *Pharmacol Rev* 55:463, 2003.
3. Oesterheld JR, Armstrong SC, Cozza KL: Ecstasy: pharmacodynamic and pharmacokinetic interactions, *Psychosomatics* 45:84, 2004.
4. Parrott AC: MDMA (3,4-methylenedioxymethamphetamine) or ecstasy: the neuropsychobiological implications of taking it at dances and raves, *Neuropsychobiology* 50:329, 2004.
5. www.drugabuse.org (An NIDA site with good information for the layperson.)
6. www.erowid.org (A website good for slang and testimonials; user must critically evaluate the information obtained from this site.)

4. Heroin

CHRISTOPHER S. RUSSI

Overview

Heroin (diacetylmorphine) is an opioid that was originally marketed in the early 1900s as a less-addictive form of morphine for pain control and a variety of disorders, from heart disease to hiccups. It is three to five times more potent than its parent drug morphine. Heroin can be administered via many routes: SQ, IM, IV, intranasal, or PO; only the most pure forms can be snorted and inhaled. It is excreted by the kidneys as morphine and 6-monoacetylmorphine (6-MAM). Opiates are the most abused class of drug in the United States, and heroin accounts for more than 90% of narcotic abuse. Often patients will "speedball" (i.e., inject the heroin with cocaine). "Chasing the dragon" refers to inhaling the vapors of heated heroin powder. This originated in Shanghai in the 1920s when porcelain bowls and bamboo tubes were used. Today, the drug is typically heated on aluminum foil and its vapors are inhaled.

Heroin and opiates are CNS depressants and will decrease pain and induce sleep. Most often the abuser is seeking a "rush" whereby the drug provides a state of euphoria or ecstasy. These drugs are chemically similar to the neurotransmitter endorphin and being highly lipophilic, the drug easily crosses to the CNS to bind the μ- and κ-opioid receptors, creating the desired effects. The serum half-life of heroin is approximately **5–9 minutes** because it is rapidly metabolized to 6-MAM. Times of peak effects and duration are variable and depend on the amount used. (See Table 9-5.) The analgesic effects generally last 3–5 hours. A dose of 5 mg of heroin is equal to 10 mg of morphine (SQ, IM) and about 1.5–2 mg of hydromorphone (Dilaudid).

Table 9-5 HEROIN KINETICS

	Onset (min)	Peak Effect (min)	Duration (min)
IV	0.1–2	10	1–240
IM	<30	5–30	Varies
Snorted/smoked	<15	5–30	Varies
SubQ		Within 90	Varies

Substances

"H," speedball (with cocaine), junk, smack, dope, hero, horse, poppy, Rambo.

See the Appendix for more street names.

Toxicity and Clinical Presentation

- You will encounter the narcotic toxidrome with overdose/ingestions.
  - Decreased BP
  - Decreased pulse rate
  - Decreased respiratory rate
  - Decreased temperature
  - Miotic pupils
- Track marks (Often, patients will develop an infection at the site of injection. Suspect drug abuse if abscesses are located around large veins.)
- Noncardiogenic pulmonary edema
  - May last 2–4 days
- Pulmonary emboli from adulterants (talc)
- Infections
  - Endocarditis
  - HIV or AIDS and hepatitis B and C
  - Lung abscess
- Rhabdomyolysis
- You will encounter opposite signs/symptoms in the **with-drawal** state.
  - Insomnia, restlessness, anxiety
  - Yawning
  - Mydriasis
  - Piloerection
  - Hyperreflexia and myoclonic jerking (known as "kicking the habit")

- Nausea and vomiting
- Abdominal cramps

Laboratory Evaluation

The following laboratory studies may be helpful in drug-related comatose patients.

- Qualitative urine drug screen
- Acetaminophen and salicylate levels
- Arterial blood gas, basic metabolic panel (do a complete metabolic panel in all comatose patients)
  - Bedside finger stick glucose
- CBC
- Liver function tests
  - May be abnormal in patients with possible hepatitis or prolonged toxicity
  - Ammonia level
  - Renal function tests, UA (urine pH may be clue to rhabdomyolysis)
- Pregnancy test in females of childbearing age
- Creatine kinase (may be clue to rhabdomyolysis)
  - Compartment syndrome can develop in these patients.
- Consider LP for cerebrospinal fluid (CSF) analysis if CNS infection is suspected.
- Radiology evaluation
  - Chest radiography
    - Noncardiogenic pulmonary typically resolves within 48 hr.
    - Consider aspiration pneumonitis or delayed acute respiratory distress syndrome (ARDS) when abnormalities develop after 48 hr.
  - Remember, adulterants may cause pulmonary abnormalities.
  - Abdominal radiographs may be helpful if you suspect that your patient is a body stuffer or packer.
  - CT scan of the brain may help to rule out brain abscesses, intracerebral or extracerebral hematomas, and stroke in the patient who is not responding to naloxone.
- EKG. Also consider an ECG because endocarditis is a common finding in IV drug abusers. You might pick up acute pulmonary hypertension (most likely due to embolic disease).

Treatment

- Anyone with altered mental status (AMS): begin with **finger-stick glucose check** and when appropriate, thiamine and oxygen.
- Treat hypoglycemia immediately.
- ABCs
- IV crystalloid for hypotension
- Give a trial of naloxone (Narcan) in suspected addicts (0.1–0.2 mg IV) or higher doses for nonaddicts (1.0–2.0 mg). Larger doses may lead to acute withdrawal symptoms.
- May be given by IV, IM, SQ, nebulized, injected submental (floor of the mouth)
- Check with friends or family; often the abuser will overdose in the company of others.

Special Considerations

Stuffers and Packers

See "Cocaine" (Special Considerations).

Pregnancy

- Can lead to miscarriage or premature birth
- Increased risk of SIDS (sudden infant death syndrome)
- Heroin crosses into breast milk and can result in sedation and respiration depression in the breast-fed infant.

Acute Opiate Withdrawal Syndrome

- Supportive care
- Clonidine can be used for autonomic symptoms.
  - 6 µg/kg acutely and 10–17 µg/kg/day (maximal dose: 25 µg/kg/day) for 10 days.
  - Watch BP for hypotension (rare, but can occur at higher doses).
  - Alternatively, 0.1–0.2 mg PO every 4 hr as needed for control of the withdrawal syndrome, for up to 7 days.
- Methadone 15–30 mg/day. **Check your state laws before administering this drug for addiction and withdrawal.**

Neonates (Neonatal Opiate Withdrawal Syndrome [NOWS])

- Can have withdrawal seizures (unlike adults, who typically do not have seizures from opiate withdrawal)
- Diazepam 1–2 mg every 8 hr. Avoid parenteral diazepam containing benzyl alcohol in jaundiced or premature infants.
- Phenobarbital should not be used alone to manage NOWS but in combination with benzodiazepines or paregoric.
  - 20 mg/kg loading dose, maintenance 2–8 mg/kg/day divided q 8–12 hr. Monitor levels daily.

Admission Criteria

- Airway protection by means of endotracheal intubation
- Altered mental status or agitation persisting for more than 4 hr in the ED after resuscitation
- Repeat dosing of naloxone required to treat severe CNS depression, slowed respirations, or hypoxia
- Iatrogenic induction of withdrawal syndrome

Pearls and Pitfalls

- Start with the low-dose naloxone in heroin addicts to avoid precipitating florid withdrawal symptoms.
  - Do not use long-acting antagonists (naltrexone) and send the patient home. These patients need to be monitored in the hospital in case they use an even larger and more dangerous amount of heroin to override the antagonist.
- Remember, you may actually see mydriasis in the **initial** phase of overdose secondary to brain hypoxia.
- Tattoos often give the drug away.
- "Chasing the dragon" originated in Shanghai in the 1920s. Porcelain bowls and bamboo tubes were used in those days. Today, the drug is typically heated on aluminum foil and the vapors are inhaled.
- The purer heroin can be snorted, and the user gets an effect similar to IV use.
- HIV or AIDS and hepatitis B and C from sharing and reusing needles and syringes for drug injection
  - Approximately one third of all HIV cases are contracted this way.

- More than 50% of all hepatitis C cases in the United States are contracted this way.
- Street adulterants such as sugar, starch, powdered milk, strychnine, and other drugs can result in further toxicity and complications.
  - Embolic phenomenon to lungs, brain, kidney
  - Seizures
  - Infection
- Withdrawal seizures typically do not occur in adults. If they are seen, think of other etiology, CNS bleed, trauma, and/or adulterant drugs that are proconvulsive.

References and Suggested Readings

1. Doyon S: Opioids. In Tintinalli J, ed: *Emergency medicine: a comprehensive study guide*, ed 6, New York, 2000, McGraw Hill, pp 1071-1075.
2. Hantsch CE, Gummin DD: Opioids. In Marx J, ed: *Rosen's emergency medicine: concepts and clinical practice*, ed 5, St Louis, 2002, Mosby, pp 2180-2187.
3. Harris CR: Opioids. In Harris CR, ed: *Emergency management of selected drugs of abuse*, Dallas, 2000, American College of Emergency Physicians, pp 77-86.
4. Kleinschmidt KC: Opioids. In Ford MD, Delaney KA, Ling LJ, Erickson T, eds: *Clinical toxicology*, Philadelphia, 2001, Saunders, pp 627-639.
5. Nelson LS: Opioids. In Goldfrank LR, eds: *Toxicologic emergencies*, ed 6, Stamford, CT, 1998, Appleton and Lange, pp 975-1000.

5. Marijuana (THC)

Marny Benjamin

Overview

Marijuana is the most commonly used illicit drug in the United States. It accounts for 77% of illegal drug use in this country. It is made from the plant *Cannabis sativa*, which can be grown indoors or outdoors. It can be smoked as a rolled cigarette paper (joint), in a pipe (bowl), or in a water pipe (bong). It can also be ingested in food such as brownies or tea.

Marijuana is used by men and women of all ethnicities and all socioeconomic classes. It is readily available in urban, suburban, and rural communities. The highest prevalence of use is among high school and college-age students. The age of first-time use is dropping every year. Between 2001 and 2003, marijuana use declined 11%, from 16.6% to 14.8%. Lifetime use declined 8.2%, from 35.3%–32.4%.

There has been a sharp increase in the number of ED visits. For youths ages 12 to 17, visits rose 126% from 1994 to 2001. For youths ages 18 to 19, the rate of marijuana-related visits increased 149% over the same time period. Some feel that this is a result of the increasing potency of marijuana available today as well as the practice of mixing it with other drugs.

Marijuana contains 421 different chemicals, 61 of which are unique to marijuana (cannabinoids). THC is thought to be the active chemical that causes the "high." In 1988, a protein receptor on nerve cells in the brain was found to bind THC. THC receptors are concentrated in the reward areas of the brain (VTA, nucleus accumbens, caudate nucleus, hippocampus) as well as other areas. The hippocampus effect explains the memory interference. Actions in the cerebellum are responsible for the disturbance in coordination and balance.

THC has been found to be psychologically addictive. *Tolerance* to the psychoactive effects develops with chronic use. Debate continues over whether there is any physical *dependence*; however, mild *withdrawal* symptoms have been reported after cessation of chronic use, including restlessness, insomnia, nausea, irritability, decreased appetite, and sweating.

Marijuana has also been mixed with methamphetamine, MDMA, prescription drugs, and ETOH. Numerous Web sites include drug slang dictionaries.

Medical uses include the treatment of asthma, nausea and vomiting associated with chemotherapy, glaucoma, spasticity, and seizures.

Rather than buying the synthetic version of THC (dronabinol or Marinol), some people grow their own from seed obtained from others or the Internet. Patients can buy 30 10-mg capsules for little more than $500.

Substances and Products

Amount of THC

The "bud"	3%–20%	
Hashish	2%–20%	Dried cannabis resin and compressed flowers
Hashish oil	15%–50%	
Average joint	1%	1% is 10 mg of THC.
Hemp	0.05%–1%	Hemp products include clothing and body care products.

Common Street Names

Weed	Grass
Pot	Dope
Mary Jane	Gonja
Doobie	Bud
Hashish	Hash
Bhang	

Street Names for Marijuana with Embalming Fluid (Formaldehyde/Methanol +/− PCP)

Fry, Fry sticks
Water-Water
Illie
Wets

Toxicity

- After smoking marijuana, effects can be felt as early as 8–9 sec. The effects peak in 10–30 min and last 1–6 hr. In 2–6 hr, users report feeling "back to normal."
- If the marijuana is eaten (cakes, cookies, and brownies are popular), the onset can be as long as 45–90 min, and its effects can last up to 12 hr.
- Marijuana is highly lipophilic and has a large volume of distribution (500 L/kg). The elimination half-life is 25–36 hr, and therefore, it stays in the system for several days.
- Higher concentrations of carbon monoxide and tar attack the respiratory system compared with smoking tobacco.
- There is 30%–50% more tar than in tobacco cigarettes. The marijuana cigarette tar contains more carcinogens than the tobacco tar.

Clinical Presentation

- See Box 9-4.
- Some patients will present with an acute psychotic reaction with hallucinations, paranoid delusions, and agitation.
  - These patients are more likely to be first-time users or to have ingested large quantities or mixed marijuana with other drugs.
- Pneumomediastinum has been described when a person holds in the smoke and then forcibly Valsalvas (tries not to laugh). It has also been reported when inhaling marijuana smoke forced into one's mouth by another's exhaling (shotgun).
- Chronic use in teenagers can lead to development of schizophrenia in adulthood.

Laboratory Evaluation

- There is no test for acute intoxication.
- Urine tests THC metabolites, which are fat soluble and can stay in the system for 3–8 weeks in chronic users and 3–10 days in sporadic users. The test can be positive as early as 30 min after use.
- False positives (rare)
  - Not seen in passive inhalation (the concertgoer)
  - NSAIDS

BOX 9-4 ▪ CLINICAL PRESENTATION OF MARIJUANA ABUSE

Acute ingestion (in order of frequency)	Chronic use
Increased heart rate	Antimotivational syndrome
Dry (cotton) mouth	Dependence (?)
Dilated pupils, conjunctival injection	Bronchitis
Relaxation	Chronic obstructive pulmonary disease (COPD)
Euphoria (the giggles)	Pharyngitis
Impaired cognitive and motor skills	Decreased fertility (men)
Hunger	Short- and long-term memory problems
Altered sensory perception	Urinary retention
Lack of motivation	Anxiety or panic
Anxiety or panic	Fantasies
Hallucinations	Hallucinations
Paranoia	Depersonalization
	Paranoia

- Ibuprofen and possibly others in the class of NSAIDs
- Efavirenz (Sustiva), the anti-HIV drug. Confirmation testing on GC/MS is typically negative.
- False negatives
  - Dilution of the urine. There is a risk of water intoxication if the person decides to dilute by drinking water rather than adding it to the urine sample.
  - Detergents, table salt, vinegar
  - Diuretic use
  - Visine: due to the benzalkonium chloride ingredient

Treatment

- Acute psychotic reaction
  - Reassurance, benzodiazepines, and time are the mainstays of treatment.

Special Considerations

- Hybrids: Users may cross-pollinate the seed and attempt to produce hybrids that contain higher concentrations of THC and thus may present with a more intense clinical picture.
- Mixing marijuana with other drugs, such as PCP, embalming fluid, or formaldehyde
- Preteens and adolescents should have social services and chemical dependency counselor involvement with their parents or guardians.

Admission Criteria

- Most adolescents can be discharged from the ED with a parent or responsible adult.
- A few hours (generally 3–6 hours) of observation in the ED is warranted to see whether the patient's symptoms clear or improve.
- Adolescents with severe intoxication may require inpatient observation overnight (12–24 hours).
- Any suspicion of neglect should be admitted for social services and notification of child protection agency.

Pearls and Pitfalls

- Urine screening tests may be positive for 3–10 days after single or sporadic use.
- Common adulterants or additives include PCP, LSD, and embalming fluid (formaldehyde and methanol). Toxicity from these drugs can cause other, more severe symptoms.
- Chronic and heavy users may have a positive urine drug screen for 3–5 weeks (sometimes longer).
- There is a strong association of early use of marijuana with developing schizophrenia as an adult.

References and Suggested Readings

1. National Institute on Drug Abuse: *NIDA InfoFacts: Marijuana.* http://www.drugabuse.gov/Infofax/marijuana.html. Accessed on March 31, 2005.
2. Otten EJ: Marijuana. In Goldfrank LR, et al, eds: *Goldfrank's toxicologic emergencies,* ed 7, New York, 2002, McGraw-Hill, pp 1054–1058.
3. Roth J: Marijuana. In Harris CR, ed: *Emergency management of selected drugs of abuse,* Dallas, 2000, American College of Emergency Physicians.

6. Mushrooms (Hallucinogenic)

CHRISTOPHER S. RUSSI

Overview

Mushrooms have been abused for many years primarily for their hallucinogenic properties. However, the desired effects can often be misplaced by the adverse effects caused by these compounds. It is *very* important that with any suspected or confirmed mushroom ingestion that one should make all attempts possible to rule out the dangerous *Amanita* species that can cause severe hepatotoxicity and death.

People who ingest mushrooms often fall into one of four major categories: (1) suicide or homicide attempts, (2) children with accidental ingestion, (3) foragers looking for edible mushrooms, and (4) abusers seeking the hallucinogenic properties.

Substances

- The most commonly abused mushroom is the *psilocybin*-containing mushroom.
- *Psilocybin:* Mushrooms of the *Psilocybe* family contain this compound and are abused and cultured primarily for their hallucinogenic effects.

Psilocybin-Containing Mushrooms Species

Psilocybe	Panaeolus	Conocybe	Gymnopilus
P. baeocystis	P. castaneifolius	C. cyanopus	G. aeruginosus
P. caerulescens	P. cyanescens	C. smithii	G. validipes
P. caerulipes	P. fimicola		
P. cyanescens	**P. foenisecii**		
P. cubensis	P. sphinctrinus		
P. pelliculosa	P. subbalteatus		
P. semilanceata			
P. strictipes			
P. stuntzii			

Common Street Names

Shrooms	Magic mushrooms
Silly putty	Sacred mushrooms
Boomers	Laughing Jim
Mushies	Little smoke
Psilocybes	Cubes
Liberty caps	Tea

Toxicity

- Resembles LSD in properties and inhibits the firing of serotonin-dependent neurons in the CNS, causing distortion of time and mood and creating hallucinations.
  - As little as 10 mg can cause euphoria and hallucinations.
  - Increasing the dose slightly will potentiate the hallucinations and cause distortion of time.
- Within 15–30 min of ingesting a muscarine mushroom, the cholinergic symptoms begin.

Clinical Presentation

- CNS: anxiety, hallucinations (more often visual than auditory), altered perception (vivid colors, kaleidoscope-like phenomenon), agitation, seizures, vertigo, paresthesias, ataxia
  - Very similar to LSD in properties
- EENT: mydriasis, tinnitus (*Panaeolus* species)
- Gastrointestinal: nausea, vomiting, mild elevation of LFTs
- Skin: facial flushing
- Symptoms begin as early as 2 hr postingestion and can last up to 4–6 hr.
- Often patients who have taken this inadvertently are quite scared.

Laboratory Evaluation

- Rule out other etiology for acute psychosis.
  - Glucose, thyroid function tests, electrolytes
  - Infectious etiology (i.e., cerebral abscess, encephalitis, cerebritis)
- Renal and hepatic function tests
- Meixner test: a bedside qualitative assay to detect amatoxins in the mushroom
  - Place a drop of freshly squeezed "juice" from the mushroom onto a piece of paper (newspaper is fine).
  - Allow it to dry or blow-dry with a low temperature setting. Then place a drop of concentrated hydrochloric acid (HCl) on the area of the mushroom drop. The area should turn blue if amatoxin is present.
  - Because false positives can occur, place another drop of HCl away from the mushroom drop as a control.

Treatment

- If the patient has AMS (altered mental status), begin by checking a finger-stick glucose and giving Narcan and, when appropriate, thiamine and oxygen.
- ABCs
- GI decontamination if the patient is willing and presents within 1 hr of ingestion
- Activated charcoal 1.0 g/kg PO

- Sedation as needed for stimulated and anxious patients: phenobarbital and benzodiazepines. **Be sure to watch the airway.**

Admission Criteria

- The altered sensorium persists after several hours in the ED, and symptoms persist after supportive care.
- The patient is critical with cholinergic symptoms requiring airway management and cardiovascular support.
- If the patient begins to develop GI symptoms including diarrhea and vomiting after 6 hr in the ED, check baseline LFTs and admit (this could be *Amanita* poisoning).
- In general, aggressive treatment is rarely necessary.

Pearls and Pitfalls

- If medics call with a mushroom poisoning, have them place the mushroom (if available) in a dry paper bag and transport it.
- Contact your state mycologist (sometimes they are at the local university) or poison control center and give details about the fungus for identification. To help the mycologist make identification, be able to provide details about:
  - Color
  - Size
  - Shape
  - Where it grew (i.e., soil or wood)
- Check if friends or family have symptoms similar to the patient.
- Do not miss hypoglycemia.

References and Suggested Readings

1. Doyon S: Opioids. In Tintinalli JE, Kelen GD, Stapczynski JS, eds: *Emergency medicine: a comprehensive study guide,* ed 6. New York, 2000, McGraw-Hill.
2. Hantsch CE, Gumminn DD: Opioids. In Marx JA, Hockberger RS, Walls RM, et al., eds: *Rosen's emergency medicine: concepts and clinical practice,* ed 5. St. Louis, 2002, Mosby.
3. Harris CR: Opioids. In Harris CR, ed: *Emergency management of selected drugs of abuse.* Dallas, 2000, American College of Emergency Physicians.

4. Nelson LS: Opioids. In Goldfrank LR, Flomenbaum NA, Lewin N, et al., eds: *Goldfrank's toxicologic emergencies*, ed 6. New York, 1998, McGraw-Hill.

5. Kleinschmidt KC: Opioids. In Ford MD, Delaney KA, Ling LJ, Erickson T, eds: *Clinical toxicology*. Philadelphia, 2001, WB Saunders.

7. Selected New Drugs of Abuse

Scott Cameron

Overview

Many drugs are abused by teens and young adults as well as a few adults. Some of these substances include inhalants, prescription narcotics, sedative/hypnotics, and nitrous oxide. A few of these drugs are reviewed here.

DEXTROMETHORPHAN

Overview

Dextromethorphan is a commonly used antitussive found in more than 140 OTC products. It is similar in structure to codeine, although it has no analgesic or addictive properties. In overdose, it produces feelings of euphoria and increased awareness with mild opioid effects. Abuse is called "robotripping," "tussing," or "robocopping." Users might be called "syrup heads" or "robotards."

It is metabolized by the P-450 system to dextrorphan, a metabolite responsible for many of the toxic effects. Duration of effect is variable and often depends on coingestants or P-450 enhancers or inhibitors; the effect generally lasts approximately 3–6 hrs.

Dextromethorphan is an NMDA antagonist, as is PCP and ketamine. Recent evidence suggests that chronic use may cause brain damage. It inhibits serotonin reuptake and may precipitate serotonin syndrome.

Substances

| Robitussin DM | Triaminic DM | Nyquil |
| Vicks pediatric formula 44 | Pediacare 1 or 3 | Coricidin |

Street Names

Dex	DM	Dextro
Robô	X	DXM
Rome	Triple Cs	Tussin
Rojo	Vitamin D	Skittles

Toxicity

- Mild intoxication (1.5–2.5 mg/kg): The first plateau is characterized by mild euphoria and is achieved with 100–250 mg of DXM (1 bottle of Robitussin DM contains 345 mg of DXM).
- Moderate intoxication (2.5–7.5 mg/kg): The second plateau has an increased euphoria, a decreased sense of time, and visual hallucinations (usually "seen" in a dark room or with the eyes closed [i.e., closed-eye visual hallucinations]). This plateau is achieved with 250–450 mg.
- Moderate severe intoxication (7.5–15 mg/kg): The third plateau is 450–800 mg and includes plateaus 1 and 2 reactions plus visual hallucinations.
- Severe intoxication is generally achieved with >15 mg/kg.
- Online calculators are available to "help" users calculate doses to attain a certain plateau.

Clinical Presentation

- Hypertension, tachycardia common
- Miosis uncommon
- Nystagmus (often vertical or rotary)
- Mild intoxication results in nausea, vomiting, ataxia, nystagmus, slurred speech, loss of coordination, and vacuous stare (hence "robotripping").
- Moderate to severe intoxication may result in seizures, stupor, tactile or auditory hallucinations, hypotension or hypertension, delusional thinking, and psychosis.
- Other unpleasant findings in the robotripper are listed in Box 9-5.

Box 9-5 ▪ Symptoms Associated with Dextromethorphan Abuse	
Nausea, vomiting, diarrhea	Dizziness
Pruritis	Blotching or flushing of the skin
Zombie walking	Ataxia
Giggling or uncontrolled laughter	Tachycardia
Respiratory depression	

Laboratory Evaluation

- None required or available for diagnosis
- Electrolytes, glucose
- Urine toxicology screen: Dextromethorphan may produce a false-positive toxicology screen for PCP.

Treatment

- Generally supportive
- GI decontamination with activated charcoal if acute presentation
- Use benzodiazepines and maintain a calm environment if patient is agitated or hypertensive.
- Response to naloxone is reported but inconsistent.
- Avoid Haldol, which lowers seizure threshold (theoretically, but why take the chance).
- Treat seizures or serotonin syndrome as necessary.

Special Considerations

- Adolescents as young as 12 years old are abusing DXM.
  - **Get help,** usually in the form of family counseling and substance abuse counseling.
- **Coricidin**
  - **Brand/Street Names:** Coricidin HBP Cold and Cough, CCC, triple C, red devils (see "Dextromethorphan" for others)
  - Coricidin HBP contains dextromethorphan hydrobromide (30 mg) and chlorpheniramine (4 mg) and is abused for the large amount of dextromethorphan in each tablet.

- Chlorpheniramine, an alkylamine antihistamine, causes anticholinergic side effects in overdose.
  - Confusion, hallucinations, agitation, hyperthermia, mydriasis, urinary retention, flushed skin
- Clinical picture is that of dextromethorphan toxicity (see "Dextromethorphan") with addition of above-listed anticholinergic effects. Bizarre behavior and hallucinations often predominate.
- Dextromethorphan hydrobromide: Chronic abuse may rarely result in bromide toxicity and negative anion gap (falsely high chloride). Symptoms include neurologic and psychiatric symptoms, rash, nausea, and vomiting.
- Management is similar to dextromethorphan.

Admission Criteria

- Most patients can be observed for 4–6 hr until effects have worn off and normal mental status is restored.
- Admit seizures, serotonin syndrome, and prolonged symptoms that make you uncomfortable (e.g., tachycardia, hypertension, or hypotension) after 6 hr of observation.

Pearls and Pitfalls

- Consider if teenager presents with vacuous stare or stupor (e.g., "robotripping" or "robocopping").
- Narcan cannot hurt and may be helpful.
- Avoid haloperidol because theoretically it may lower the seizure threshold.
- "Agent Lemon Extraction Method" is a means of extracting dextromethorphan from the syrup or pills. This method uses household ammonia, Zippo lighter fluid, and lemon juice.
- Users will try to attain 1 of 4 plateaus by taking a certain number of pills or drinking a certain amount of syrup. To calculate the dose, a "calculator" found on several Internet sites can be used online or downloaded to the user's computer.
- Serotonin syndrome can be precipitated, especially when combined with serotonergic drugs/medications.
- False positive for PCP
- Coricidin HBP abusers may present with elevated chloride and bromide toxicity.

References and Suggested Readings

1. Banerji S, Anderson I: Abuse of Coricidin HBP cough & cold: episodes recorded by a poison center, *Am J Health Syst Pharm* 58:1811, 2001.
2. Boyer EW: Dextromethorphan abuse [Review], *Ped Emerg Care* 20:858, 2004.
3. DXM. http://www.erowid.org/chemicals/dxm/dxm.shtml. Accessed May 20, 2003.
4. National Drug Intelligence Center: "Triple C" fast facts, 2003, Department of Justice. Available at http://www.usdoj.gov/ndic/pub6/6906. Accessed May 20, 2003.
5. Wolfe TR, Caravati EM: Massive dextromethorphan ingestion and abuse, *Am J Emerg Med* 13:174, 1995.

OXYCONTIN

Overview

OxyContin contains oxycodone, a synthetic opioid used for chronic and severe pain. It is usually crushed and snorted or injected, producing a rapid onset of euphoria and a "heroin-like" high. It is sometimes referred to as "hillbilly heroin" or "poor man's heroin." It is available in doses up to 160 mg (compared with 5 mg for Vicodin). The street value is approximately $1/mg. It has a high potential for abuse and has rapidly become a leading drug of abuse on the East Coast. A large proportion of crime in many communities is attributed to OxyContin. It was originally thought to have a low potential for abuse due to the slow release of oxycodone.

Recently, manufacturers have taken steps to stem abuse, including the removal of the highest doses and reformulation with microencapsulated naloxone that is released only if the capsule is crushed for snorting or injection.

Substances and Street Names

Oxy, OC, Os, poor man's heroin, hillbilly heroin

Toxicity

- OxyContin abusers have a greater risk of death when they combine alcohol or other CNS depressants.

- Some abusers crush the pills and inject the medication IV. Needless to say, their toxicity is increased, and they may present in severe respiratory depression, acute pulmonary edema, or death.

Clinical Presentation

- Opioid agonist, causes opioid toxicity
- Causes typical opioid toxidrome: miosis, decreased mental status, and respiratory depression
- Drowsiness, euphoria, and conjunctival injection are also common.
- Like all "good" opioids, may cause noncardiogenic pulmonary edema

Laboratory Evaluation

Diagnosis is often made on empiric treatment with naloxone and history. Toxicology screening is helpful for the psychiatrist, and the law, and the lab Christmas party fund.

Treatment

- Maintain patent airway, assist ventilation, O_2, IV, monitor.
- Early use of naloxone may obviate need for intubation in severe cases.
  - Start with 0.4–2.0 mg IV. Up to 10–20 mg may be required for large overdoses; may require drip.
  - Naloxone lasts 1–2 hr. Oxycontin lasts 4–6 hr. All but trivial intoxications require at least 6 hr of observation.
  - Start naloxone drip if severe/refractory respiratory depression (also consider other diagnosis). Give two thirds of initial waking naloxone dose over 1 hr.
- Consider activated charcoal (after naloxone) if airway is secure and clinical picture warrants it.

Admission Criteria and Disposition

- Observe any symptomatic patient for at least 6 hr.
- Admit any patient requiring administration of naloxone and any patient with unstable vital signs or pulmonary edema.

Pearls and Pitfalls

- Put on the restraints before naloxone administration (if not in extremis, obviously).
- Miosis, CNS, and respiratory depression equal opiate overdose.
- Some predict that OxyContin could outstrip cocaine as the no. 1 drug of abuse.

References and Suggested Reading

1. Cone EJ, Fant RV, Rohay JM, et al: Oxycodone involvement in drug abuse deaths. II. Evidence for toxic multiple drug-drug interactions, *J Anal Toxicol* 28:217, 2004.
2. Government Accounting Office: OxyContin abuse and diversion and efforts to address the problem: highlights of a government report, *J Pain Palliat Care Pharmacother* 18:109, 2004.
3. Meadows M: Prescription drug use and abuse. http://www.fda.gov/fdac/features/2001/501_drug.html. Accessed Dec 4, 2004.

Chapter 10

Date-Rape Drugs

CARSON R. HARRIS

▉ Overview

The incidence of drug-facilitated sexual assault is definitely increasing. The drug most commonly associated with sexual assault is ethanol, but other drugs, also known as "club drugs" because of their popularity in dance clubs and rave bars, can be unknowingly given to a victim. The effect sought is to incapacitate and prevent the victim from resisting during a sexual assault or other crime. These drugs can also produce amnesia, causing a victim to be unclear of what, if any, crime was committed and unable to identify the attacker. This fear of the unknown can amplify the victim's trauma symptoms. Acquaintance or date rape is severely underreported.

▉ Substances

Common Sedatives/Hypnotics, Anesthetics, or CNS Depressants with Their Street Names	
Gamma-hydroxybutyrate (GHB)	G, G-riffic, liquid ecstasy, liquid X, easy lay, cherry meth
Ketamine	K, vitamin K, special K
Flunitrazepam (Rohypnol)	Roofies, roach, ropes, R-2
Clonazepam	

■ Toxicity

- The dangers of date-rape drugs
  - When combined with alcohol may lead to respiratory depression and death
  - Coma, aspiration, seizure, anoxic brain injury
  - Victims unable to protect themselves from HIV, other sexually transmitted diseases (STDs), or unintended pregnancy

■ Clinical Presentation

- Amnesia, especially short term with difficulty retrieving information related to the assault
  - Amnesia consisting of a several-hour gap in the memory of the previous night
- Decreased inhibition
- CNS depression
- Generally, by the time the victim arrives to the ED, most signs and symptoms have resolved.
- Hallucination- or nightmare-like event upon awakening (ketamine)
- Respiratory arrest
- Aspirations
- Seizure, coma, death (the **final** common pathway)

■ Laboratory Evaluation

- GHB is the most common drug used to facilitate sexual assault, and unfortunately it has a very short half-life. Thus, the yield for positive tests of GHB in urine is relatively low.
- Depending on the dose, some benzodiazepines may remain in the urine for 2–3 days. However, the typical urine drug screen will miss the newer benzodiazepines, and a comprehensive screen should be requested with a specific request for the suspected benzodiazepines. Clonazepam typically yields a false-negative rapid urine drug screen.
- Some institutions have a "date-rape panel" that tests for the commonly used drugs in sexual assault (GHB, flunitrazepam, ethanol, barbiturates, benzodiazepine, and ketamine).

- For GHB, the best time period for sampling urine is 3–10 hr postingestion.
- For Rohypnol and short-acting barbiturates, the best time for sampling is within 24 hr postingestion (Table 10-1).
- Evidentiary exams should be performed by practitioners with specific knowledge regarding evidence collection and chain of custody.

Treatment

- Supportive care is recommended. See Chapter 4, Benzodiazepines.
- Counseling by qualified personnel
- Manage traumatic injuries as necessary and with caution so as to not disturb evidence.
- Treat for presumptive STDs (e.g., chlamydia, GC, syphilis).

Table 10-1 DETECTION IN URINE

	DETECTION IN URINE	
Drug	**Acute Use**	**Chronic Use**
Amphetamines	1 day	Several weeks
Barbiturates	Short acting (e.g., secobarbital): 1 day	
	Long acting (e.g., phenobarbital): 2–3 weeks	
Benzodiazepines	3 days	4–6 weeks
Cocaine metabolites	2–3 days	Several days
Codeine/morphine	2–4 days	Several days
GHB	3–10 hr	Up to 12–24 hr
Methadone	2–3 days	1–2 weeks
PCP	Up to 1 week	1–2 weeks
Propoxyphene	1–2 days	Several days
Marijuana	Single smoke: up to 4 days	
	Moderate use: up to 10 days	
	Heavy use: up to 4–6 weeks	
	Passive inhalation (e.g., concertgoer): negative	
Nicotine	Moderate use: 1–2 days	

Adapted from http://www.emedhome.com/resources/pdfdatabase/27.pdf. Accessed Dec 4, 2004.

■ Special Considerations

- Trauma
- STDs
- Psychological trauma and depression

■ Admission Criteria

- Altered mental status after 6-hr observation period
- Signs of aspiration
- Significant depression and suicidal ideations

Pearls and Pitfalls

- Most cases do not require admission.
- Physostigmine for GHB should be used with great caution.
- A woman may want to collect a sample of her urine in a clean container and place in the refrigerator if she **suspects** that she may have been drugged. That sample can be brought to the ED or her physician once she **decides** to be evaluated (preferably within 48 hr of the suspected assault).
- Review your hospital's or department's protocol or policy for managing sexual assaults.

■ References and Suggested Readings

1. Drug Detection Time in Urine Following Last Dose. SOURCE: Quest Diagnostics, Cambridge, Massachusetts.http://www.emedhome.com/resources/pdfdatabase/27. pdf. Accessed Dec. 4, 2004.
2. Groulle JP, Anger JP: Drug-facilitated robbery or sexual assault: problems associated with amnesia. *Ther Drug Monit* 2004;26(2):206–210.

Chapter 11

Toxic Alcohols

James Winter

1. Methanol

Overview

Methanol, also known as wood alcohol or methyl alcohol, has uses as a solvent in varnishes and chemical syntheses and is commonly used as antifreeze in windshield washer fluids. It is the denaturant in denatured alcohol. A large number of deaths have occurred as it was made or substituted for ethanol. Methanol's distribution is wide, and it is metabolized and excreted slower than ethanol (i.e., at about 20% of the rate of ethanol). Formic acid is the principle cause of toxicity, involving most of the anion gap (lactic acid also contributes to this), metabolic acidosis, and ocular toxicity. Methanol inhibits cytochrome oxidase in the ocular fundi. Swelling of axons in the optic disc and edema result in visual impairment. Degradation of formic acid is folate dependent. Thus if a folate-deficient person ingests ethanol, toxicity may be more severe due to the increased accumulation of formic acid.

Substances

Colonial spirit	Columbian spirit(s)	***Methyl alcohol***
Methyl hydroxide	Methylol	Monohydroxymethane
Purple lady (slang term) – 5% methanol and 90% ethanol	Pyroxylic spirit	***Wood alcohol***
Wood naphtha	***Wood spirit***	

Sources

Windshield wiper fluid	Paints	**Varnish removers**
Industrial solvent	Manufacture of formaldehyde and acetic acid	***Antifreeze***
Fuel anti-icing additive	Fuel octane booster	***Sterno*** (fuel for picnic stoves
Soldering torches	Ethanol denaturant	Extractant solvent

Methanol is also used as a solvent in the manufacture of cholesterol, streptomycin, vitamins, hormones, and other pharmaceuticals.

Toxicity

$$\text{Methanol} \rightarrow \text{Formaldehyde} \rightarrow \text{Formic Acid} \rightarrow CO_2 + H_2O$$

- Metabolized in the liver (90%–95%), primarily by alcohol and aldehyde dehydrogenase
  - Formate inhibits cytochrome oxidase affecting mitochondrial respiration and reduction in glutathione concentration. This also results in lactate formation and oxidative stress in the retina.
  - Formaldehyde has a short half-life, lasting only minutes.
  - Formic acid is metabolized much more slowly, and it bioaccumulates with significant methanol ingestion.
- Toxicity is due primarily to formic acid or formaldehyde affecting retinal cells.
- The total fatal dose is the subject of some controversy, but it is thought to be as little as 50 mL or 1 mL/kg.

Clinical Presentation

- Poisoning with methanol presents with intoxication, headache, fatigue, nausea, and potential visual blurring.
- With increasing dose, all the above worsen, with vomiting as well as CNS depression occurring.
- Visual disturbance can then become profound (e.g., haziness or whiteout), with permanent loss of vision after days. Optic disc hyperemia can occur.
- Severe symptoms include respiratory depression, coma, hypotension, severe acidosis, and death.
  - 0–20 mg/dL: Usually asymptomatic
  - 20–50 mg/dL: Generally requires treatment
  - +150 mg/dL: Potentially fatal if untreated
- Other systems affected represent **chronic intoxication** concerns and should be considered (Box 11-1).

Laboratory Evaluation

- Electrolytes, BUN, and creatinine
  - Serum bicarbonate will be very low (i.e., in the low teens or lower).
  - High anion gap metabolic acidosis
- Glucose: Hypoglycemia can occur.

BOX 11-1 ▪ CLINICAL EFFECTS OF METHANOL POISONING

Neuropsychiatric

Withdrawal, hallucinations, excitation, neuropathy

Gastrointestinal

Gastritis, fatty liver, cirrhosis, pancreatitis

Cardiovascular

Cardiomyopathy, hypertension

Pulmonary

Pneumonia, aspirations

Hematologic and metabolic

Anemias, acidosis, hypoglycemia, hyperuricemia, hyperlipidemia, hyperamylasemia

- CBC to evaluate for anemia
- ABG
  - Severe acidosis is a bad prognostic sign.
- A blood methanol level is possible to obtain in many laboratories with the level of 20 mg/dL significant. The level of 40 mg/dL is generally an indication of serious poisoning and requires therapy or hemodialysis.
- Serum formic acid levels (a great predictor of toxicity) could be useful, but presently, results are not timely enough to affect management.
- Serum osmolality
  - Calculate osmol gap (measured osmols – calculated osmols)
    - The most commonly used formula: $(2 \times Na) + (BUN \div 2.8) + (Glu \div 18)$
    - A gap of more than 50 mOsm/L is most likely caused by a toxic alcohol ingestion.
    - Normal gap does not exclude toxic alcohol ingestion.
- Urine assay
- The patient's urine may have an odor of formaldehyde.

Treatment

Large volumes of acutely ingested methanol may be lavaged. If Antizol (Jazz Pharmaceuticals, Palo Alto, CA) is not available, a call to the regional poison center will assist the practitioner in the initiation of an ethanol infusion or oral intake of 100-proof ethanol at 1.5 to 2.0 mL/kg with infusion.

- Fomepizole (Antizol) treatment has been used and can be guided by the Regional Poison Center.
  - 15 mg/kg loading dose over 30 min, followed by 10 mg/kg q 12 hr × 4 doses; then, if necessary, 15 mg/kg q 12 hr until methanol level <20 mg/dL
    - The increase in maintenance doses from 10 mg/kg to 15 mg/kg is due to the autoinduction of fomepizole metabolism.
- Monitor the acidosis early and often; if it is sustained, hemodialysis may be entertained.
  - Sodium bicarbonate
- Administer thiamine and folate as cofactor enhancements.
  - Folate: The precise dose is unknown, but 50 mg IV every 4 hr for 24 hr should be given as soon as methanol ingestion is suspected. Folate (or its active form, folinic acid) enhances the metabolism of formate to CO_2 and water.

- Maintain adequate urinary output and central monitoring.
- Hemodialysis is indicated if failure of treatment and increasing acidosis or hemodynamic instability.
  - Severe acidosis (i.e., pH <7.20) not responding to your treatment
  - Methanol serum concentrations more than 50 mg/dL
  - Renal failure
  - Visual symptoms
- Ethanol can be administered PO or IV (best method of administration).
- Loading dose: 0.8 gm/kg of a 10% solution infused over 1 hr

See Table 11-1.

Special Considerations

- Pediatric ingestions
  - Toxic alcohols should be considered in the child with altered mental status of unknown cause. The child may have ingested a product containing a toxic alcohol (i.e., radiator antifreeze that was placed in a soda bottle or sports drink bottle).

Admission Criteria

- CNS depression
- Acidosis

Table 11-1	ETHANOL INFUSION TREATMENT FOR METHANOL AND ETHYLENE GLYCOL POISONING				
	Dose Ranges in mg/kg/hr	**Infusion Rates in ml/hr for Various Patient Weights**			
		10 kg	**30 kg**	**70 kg**	**100 kg**
Normal maintenance	80	8	24	56	80
	110	11	33	77	110
	130	13	39	91	130
Alcoholics	150			105	150
During dialysis	250	25	75	175	250
	300	30	90	210	300
	350	35	105	245	350

Adapted from Howland MA: Antidotes in depth. Ethanol. In Goldfrank LR, Hoffman RS, Lewin NA, eds, et al: Goldfrank's toxicologic emergencies, ed 7, New York, 2002, McGraw-Hill.

- Level greater than 20 mg/dL with altered mental status and/or acidosis
- Abnormal eye findings or complaint of visual disturbance

Pearls and Pitfalls

- A negative methanol level in an apparently intoxicated patient with severe acidosis does not preclude methanol poisoning.
- A formate level may be the clue, but it generally takes several days to get the results.
- Monitor the electrolytes and blood sugar carefully.
- Do not forget about the treatment of alcohol withdrawal syndromes, especially seizures, and the use of benzodiazepines for treatment.
- Beware of the alcoholic transferred from Detox who is "not waking up as usual." The patient may have ingested a toxic alcohol.
- Social services referral for poison prevention, home monitoring if children are involved, and referral for substance abuse counseling are warranted.
- Beware of possible head trauma and intracranial bleed. Order a CT scan of the head for suspected trauma.

References and Suggested Readings

1. Alcohols and glycols. In Ellenhorn MJ, Schonwald S, Ordog G, Wasserberger J, eds: *Ellenhorn's medical toxicology: diagnosis and treatment of human poisoning.* Baltimore, 1997, Williams & Wilkins, pp 1127–1165.

2. Barceloux DG, Bond GR, Krenzelok EP, et al. American Academy of Clinical Toxicology practice guidelines on the treatment of methanol poisoning, *J Toxicol Clin Toxicol* 40:415–446, 2002.

3. Egland AG, Landry DR: *Alcohols, toxicity.* http://www.emedicine.com/emerg/topic19.htm. Last updated Apr 24, 2002. Accessed Dec 5, 2004.

4. Ford MD, McMartin K: Ethylene glycol and methanol. In Ford MD, Delaney KA, Ling LJ, Erickson T, eds: *Clinical toxicology,* Philadelphia, 2001, WB Saunders, pp 757–768.

5. Howland MA: Antidotes in depth. Ethanol. In Goldfrank LR, Flomenbaum NA, Lewin N, eds, et al: *Goldfrank's toxicologic emergencies,* ed 7, New York, 2002, McGraw-Hill, pp 1064–1066.

6. MICROMEDEX® Healthcare Series, vol 123. Expired March 2005. Accessed Dec 5, 2004.

7. Olson KR, Anderson IB, Benowitz NL, et al, eds: *Poisoning and drug overdose,* ed 4. New York, 2003, McGraw-Hill.

8. Schonwald S: *Medical toxicology: a synopsis and study guide,* 2001, Lippincott, Williams & Wilkins, pp 162–165.

2. Ethylene Glycol

Overview

Ethylene glycol (EG) toxicity must be recognized early, and treatment must be initiated in a rapid and aggressive manner to prevent death. EG has a sweet taste and is generally well tolerated initially during consumption in poisoning. It is widely distributed in the body and is metabolized to oxalic acid, which is thought to cause its damaging effects in overdose.

Substances

- The principle ingredient in antifreeze and many types of brake fluids
  - More than 25% of the ethylene glycol produced is used in antifreeze and coolant mixtures for motor vehicles.
  - Used in aircraft deicing
  - Used in condensers and heat exchangers
- Commonly used to mark centerlines of roads and runways during snow and ice periods
- Also used as a solvent and an industrial humectant
- Used as a chemical intermediate to produce polyester fibers, films, and resins and as a glycerin substitute in commercial products such as paints, lacquers, detergents, and cosmetics

Toxicity

- Brain injury as well as renal injury can occur, with calcium oxalate crystals being found in organs such as the spinal cord, kidneys, and brain.
- Acute poisoning of EG is an amount generally over 100 mL in a single dose; however, lower amounts have caused considerable risk.
- The fatal dose of EG is debatable but is thought to be approximately 50–100 g.
- Death may occur early from respiratory failure.

Clinical Presentation

- Symptoms are those of any alcohol intoxication but may progress to vomiting, cyanosis, tachycardia, tachypnea, stupor, respiratory distress, coma, and seizures.

- Hypocalcemia tetany can occur due to the precipitation of calcium in crystal formation. Hemolysis can occur.
- Some patients may present with severe metabolic acidosis with high anion and osmolal gaps, plus calcium oxalate crystals in the urine.
- Three stages of toxicity (Table 11-2)
  - **Remember, the patient can present in any stage.**
    - Renal failure may appear early in severe poisonings and progress to anuria. Hematuria and proteinuria are common. In surviving cases, renal function usually returns to normal, but permanent renal damage has occurred in some cases. Serious hepatic injury is uncommon.

Table 11-2 THREE STAGES OF TOXICITY

Stages	Timing Postingestion (hrs)	Presentation
Stage 1: Neurologic	0.5–12	Transient inebriation, euphoria
		Nausea, vomiting (results of direct gastric irritation)
		Coma or seizures, meningismus
		Metabolic acidosis, CNS depression from toxic metabolites (usually 4–12 hr postingestion)
		Papilledema may be seen (check for it).
Stage 2: Cardiopulmonary	12–24	Tachycardia, hypertension
		Severe metabolic acidosis
		Compensatory hyperventilation
		Hypoxia
		Congestive heart failure
		Acute respiratory distress syndrome
		Most deaths occur in Stage 2 from multiple organ failure.
Stage 3: Renal	24–72	Oliguria
		Acute tubular necrosis
		Renal failure
		Hematuria, proteinuria
		Bone marrow suppression occurs during Stage 3.

Laboratory Evaluation

- UA must be attained and examined for calcium oxalate crystals. The examiner may see red blood cells (RBCs) and casts in the urine.
  - The absence of calcium oxalate crystals does not rule out EG ingestion.
- Electrolytes, glucose, BUN/Cr, calcium, anion gap
  - Hyperkalemia may occur with hypocalcemia.
  - Serum bicarbonate will be low.
  - Calculate serum osmols.
- Measure serum osmols and calculate osmolar gap.
  - Increased osmolal gap
    - High osmolal gap with low ethylene glycol levels may be due to persistent glycolate in plasma.
    - But remember, a low or normal osmolal gap does not rule out EG poisoning.
    - Normal osmolal gap may be an indication that the patient has metabolized most of the compound.
- A serum EG may be obtained.
  - Generally, a level over 50 mg/dL is considered significant and life-threatening.
- ABGs
- Head CT to rule out head trauma or other etiology for altered mental status (AMS)
- CBC

Treatment

- Large volumes of acutely ingested ethylene glycol may be lavaged if the patient arrives within 30 min of ingestion.
- Pyridoxine 50 mg IV q 6 hr for 2 days as cofactor support
  - In the presence of magnesium, pyridoxine drives the metabolism of glyoxalate to the harmless glycine metabolite.
- Thiamine 100 mg IV q 6 hr for 2 days as cofactor support
  - In the presence of magnesium, thiamine drives the metabolism of glyoxalate to α-OH-β-ketoadipate, thereby decreasing the production of oxalic acid (the "bad stuff").
- Antizol treatment has been used and can be guided by the Regional Poison Center.
  - Fomepizole is a competitive inhibitor of alcohol dehydrogenase and effectively blocks toxic metabolite formation.

- Dose: 15 mg/kg loading dose followed by 10 mg/kg IV dose q 12 hr for four doses, then 15 mg/kg q 12 hr until level is below 20 mg/dL
- Give q 4 hr if dialyzing the patient.
- If fomepizole (Antizol) is not available, a call to the Regional Poison Center will assist the practitioner in the initiation of an ethanol infusion or oral intake of 100-proof ethanol at 1.5–2.0 mL/kg with infusion.
  - For ethanol treatment, see "Methanol."
- Monitor the acidosis early and often; if it is sustained, hemodialysis may be entertained.
- Maintain adequate urinary output and central monitoring.
- Give calcium gluconate, 10 mL of 10% CaGlu in D5W, to maintain serum calcium levels.
- Hemodialysis is indicated if acidosis fails to respond to treatment and/or shows increased hemodynamic instability (Box 11-2).

Special Considerations

Chronic Intoxication

- May present with neuropsychiatric syndromes of withdrawal, hallucinations, excitation, neuropathy; gastrointestinal symptoms of gastritis, fatty liver, cirrhosis, pancreatitis; cardiovascular syndromes of cardiomyopathy, hypertension; pulmonary symptoms of pneumonia, aspirations; hematologic and metabolic symptoms of anemia, acidosis, hypoglycemia, hyperuricemia, hyperlipidemia, hyperamylasemia.

Admission Criteria

- Any patient requiring antidote treatment
- Abnormal CNS
- Suicidal

BOX 11-2 ■ HEMODIALYSIS INDICATIONS	
• Acidosis failing to respond to adequate bicarbonate treatment	• Increase in creatinine of ≥1 mg/dL (88 mmol/L)
• Serum creatinine >3 mg/dL (265 µmol/L)	• Initial ethylene glycol ≥50 mg/dL (8.1 mmol/L)

- Chronic alcoholic with suspicion for ingestion of EG and with altered mental status
- Metabolic acidosis and suspicion of toxic alcohol ingestion

Pearls and Pitfalls

- A negative EG level is not necessarily proof of noningestion of EG.
- An acidosis with crystalloid may be indicative enough to begin the treatment course.
- Maintain urine output.
- Monitor the electrolytes and blood sugar carefully.
- Do not forget about the treatment of alcohol withdrawal syndromes, especially seizures, and the use of benzodiazepines for treatment.
- Social services referral for poison prevention, home monitoring if children are involved, and referral for substance abuse counseling are warranted.
- CNS depression in pediatric patients may be due to alcohol-induced hypoglycemia.
- A low or normal osmolal gap does not rule out the diagnosis of EG poisoning.

References and Suggested Readings

1. Alcohol and glycols. In Ellenhorn MJ, Schonwald S, Ordog G, Wasserberger J, eds: *Medical toxicology: diagnosis and treatment of human poisoning*, ed 2. Baltimore, 1997, Williams & Wilkins.
2. Barceloux DG, Krenzelok EP, Olson KR, Watson M: American Academy of Clinical Toxicology practice guidelines on the treatment of ethylene glycol poisoning, *J. Toxicol Clin Toxicol* 37:537–560, 1999.
3. Ethylene glycol. In Olson KR, Anderson IB, Benowitz NL, et al, eds: *Poisoning and drug overdose*, ed 4. New York, 2003, McGraw-Hill.
4. Ethylene, propylene, and diethylene glycol. In Schonwald S: *Medical toxicology: a synopsis and study guide*. Philadelphia, 2001, Lippincott, Williams & Wilkins, pp 165–167.
5. Ford MD, McMartin K: Ethylene glycol and methanol. In Ford MD, Delaney KA, Ling LJ, Erickson T, eds: *Clinical toxicology*, Philadelphia, 2001, WB Saunders, pp 757–768.
6. Goldfrank LR, Flomenbaum NE: Toxic alcohols. In Goldfrank LR, Hoffman RS, Lewin NA, et al, eds: *Goldfrank's toxicologic emergencies*, ed. 7. New York, 2002, McGraw-Hill, pp 1049–1070.
7. Micromedex Healthcare Series, vol 123, expired June 2006. Accessed Dec 5, 2004.

3. Isopropyl Alcohol

Overview

Isopropanol is generally thought of as rubbing alcohol. Its common household uses include shaving lotions, aftershaves, cleaners, and window cleaners, and it is used in industry for general purposes. It is more toxic than ethanol; about 250 mL is considered a fatal dose. Between 50% and 80% of isopropanol is metabolized to acetone. The rest is excreted, unchanged, by the kidneys. Acetone is excreted by the kidneys primarily and also by the lungs. The elimination half-life of isopropanol is 4–6 hours. The elimination half-life of acetone is about 16–20 hours.

Substances

"Rub-a-dub" is the street name for rubbing alcohol (70% isopropyl alcohol).

Toxicity

- About 250 mL is considered a fatal dose.
- Fatal cases show pulmonary involvement of bronchitis, edema, and hemorrhage.

Clinical Presentation

- CNS depression is the key hallmark of isopropanol intoxication.
- The patient will appear intoxicated but has the odor of acetone on the breath instead of ethanol (distilled spirits).
- Persistent complications exceed those of ethanol intoxication and include abdominal pain, tenderness, hemorrhage, marked respiratory depression, and CNS depression leading to coma, areflexia, and death (Box 11-3).
- Prolonged CNS toxicity is due in part to acetone.
  - Other affected systems represent chronic intoxication concerns and should be considered
  - Neuropsychiatric syndromes of withdrawal, hallucinations, excitation, neuropathy

BOX 11-3 ■ SYMPTOMS OF ISOPROPYL ALCOHOL TOXICITY

Neurologic

CNS depression, coma
Ataxia
Slurred speech
Loss of deep tendon reflexes may be noted

EENT

Nystagmus, miosis

GI

Abdominal pain
Nausea, vomiting
Hematemesis
Gastritis, hemorrhagic gastritis

Cardiovascular

Hypotension (secondary to vasodilation, negative inotropic effects)
Sinus tachycardia

Respiratory

Respiratory depression
Pulmonary edema in fatal cases (rare)

Other systems

Acute tubular necrosis (rare), myoglobinuria
Hepatic dysfunction (rare)
Hemolytic anemia (rare)

- Gastrointestinal symptoms of gastritis, fatty liver, cirrhosis, pancreatitis
- Cardiovascular syndromes of cardiomyopathy, hypertension
- Pulmonary symptoms of pneumonias, aspirations
- Hematologic and metabolic symptoms of anemias, acidosis, hypoglycemia, hyperuricemia, hyperlipidemia, hyperamylasemia
- Metabolic acidosis is **not** a finding of isopropanol, unlike the other toxic alcohols. Because the end product of isopropanol is acetone and acetone is a ketone, it does not typically cause metabolic acidosis.

Laboratory Evaluation

- Urinalysis, basic chemistry panel, liver enzymes, CBC
  - Acetonemia and acetonuria with hypoglycemia are keys to the diagnosis with the clinical presentation.
  - Elevated BUN and liver enzymes can be found with an ongoing anemia due to hemolysis.
- Serum osmols
- Isopropyl alcohol level
- Other tests appropriate for patient presentation
  - Head CT scan
  - Chest radiograph
  - Lumbar pressure

Treatment

- Provide supportive care with detail to renal involvement.
- Monitor sugars closely and treat hypoglycemia.
- Monitor the hematocrit closely.
- Isopropyl alcohol rarely requires antidote or hemodialysis treatment.

Special Considerations

- Consider trauma, especially of the head. Search the patient for telltale trauma findings on the head, trunk, and extremities.
- Seizures or postictal state
  - Consider other etiologies for seizures (see "Mnemonics" for toxic seizures).
  - Pediatric ingestion
- Do not forget to remind the parent to keep all medications and chemicals out of the child's reach or locked in a secure cabinet.

Admission Criteria

- Admit patients with any of the following:
  - CNS depression
  - Hypotension

- Electrolyte abnormalities requiring interventions
- Discharge the hemodynamically stable patient who is not obtunded after 6 hr postingestion.

Pearls and Pitfalls

- Recovery is usually complete if supportive care is detailed.
- Treat the renal involvement.
- Symptoms may last longer (e.g., days) than with ethanol intoxication.
- Do not forget about the treatment of alcohol withdrawal syndromes, especially seizures, and the use of benzodiazepines for treatment.
- Social services referral for poison prevention, home monitoring if children are involved, and referral for substance abuse counseling are warranted.
- Remember, the population that is most often seen and admitted for isopropyl ingestion is the chronic alcoholic who is subject to numerous disease processes and trauma (e.g., meningitis, intracranial bleeding, pneumonia, sepsis, seizures, hypoglycemia, alcohol ketoacidosis).

References and Suggested Readings

1. Alcohol and glycols. In Ellenhorn MJ, Schonwald S, Ordog G, Wasserberger J, eds: *Medical toxicology: diagnosis and treatment of human poisoning*, ed 2, Baltimore, 1997, Williams & Wilkins.
2. Ford MD: Isopropanol. In Ford MD, Delaney KA, Ling LJ, Erickson T, eds: *Clinical toxicology*, Philadelphia, 2001, WB Saunders, pp 769–773.
3. Goldfrank LR, Flomenbaum NE: Toxic alcohols. In Goldfrank LR, Holfman RS, Lewin NA, et al, eds: *Goldfrank's toxicologic emergencies*, ed. 7, New York, 2002, McGraw-Hill, pp 1049–1070.
4. Isopropyl alcohol. In Olson KR, Anderson IB, Benowitz NL, et al, eds: *Poisoning and drug overdose*, ed 4, New York, 2003, McGraw-Hill.
5. Isopropyl alcohol. In Schonwald S: *Medical toxicology: a synopsis and study guide*, Philadelphia, 2001, Lippincott, Williams & Wilkins.

Chapter 12

Metals: Arsenic, Lead, Mercury, and Metal Fume Fever

Beth Baker and Michael McGrail

▨ Overview

Arsenic

Arsenic is a well-known poison that has been used throughout history. Arsenic exposure may occur through intentional poisoning or contaminated drinking water (a worldwide problem). Arsenic is tasteless and odorless and is well absorbed by the respiratory or gastrointestinal tract (Box 12-1).

Lead

Lead poisoning or plumbism is a particular concern in children. The Centers for Disease Control and Prevention recommends universal screening of children for lead poisoning and community intervention if the child's blood lead level (BLL) is equal to or >10 μg/dL. BLLs declined 78% overall in the United States between 1976 and 1991 due to better environmental controls, banning of lead-based residential paint, and regulated removal of leaded gasoline[2] (Box 12-2).

Mercury

Mercury was used in the felt industry, and patients with mercury poisoning were labeled "Mad Hatters." Mercury-contaminated

Box 12-1 ▪ Potential Sources of Arsenic Exposure[1]

Intentional poisoning	Arsenical pesticides
Rock and volcanic eruptions	Contaminated drinking water
Organic arsenic from eating fish or seafood	Gallium arsenide used in computer and semiconductor
Arsenic containing wood preservatives	Arsine gas
Smelting of metals	Opium

Box 12-2 ▪ Sources of Lead Poisoning[3,4]

Leaded paint in older homes or commercial sites	Ethnic fold remedies such as azarcon, greta
Industrial waste	Drinking water
Automobile exhaust	Soil and dust
Remodeling of structures with lead-based paints	Lead battery manufacturers or recyclers
Lead solder	Lead smelters
Lead refiners	Tetraethyl lead
Lead-based pigments and stabilizers	Lead-glazed ceramics
Leaded ammunition	

fish is a concern throughout the world. Organic mercury or methylmercury bioaccumulates in the food chain and thus large predatory fish such as **shark, swordfish, king mackerel,** and **tilefish** have higher mercury levels than do small fish[5] (Box 12-3).

Metal Fume Fever

Metal fume fever is a self-limiting, acute illness that occurs after exposure to metal oxide fumes. It results in flulike symptoms (Box 12-4).

Substances

- Arsenic, lead, mercury, zinc, chromium, iron, magnesium, brass
- 70% of the world's production of arsenic is used as copper chrome arsenate (CCA) as a wood preservative.
- 22% of the world's arsenic production is used as pesticides in agricultural chemicals.
- The remainder is used in metallurgy, glass, and pharmaceuticals.

BOX 12-3 ■ **SOURCES OF MERCURY EXPOSURE[6,7]**

Food or grain treated with fungicides
   containing mercury
Dental amalgams[*]
Thimerosal (preservative that contains
   ethylmercury)
Disc batteries

Fish from contaminated bodies
   of water
Amalgam makers
Mercury thermometers
Dyes

---

[*]*Most experts do not believe that this can cause significant symptoms; however, there is not universal agreement on this topic.*

BOX 12-4 ■ **SOURCES OF EXPOSURE[8,9]**

Welding of mercury, zinc, chromium,
   or galvanized iron
Zinc smelting
Magnesium fumes
Molten metal fabricators
Steel alloy manufacturers

Bronzing, galvanizing, casting,
   brazing
Brass foundry workers
Brass solderers
Metal grinders

▌ Toxicity

Arsenic

- Multiple forms: elemental, inorganic, organic, arsine gas, trivalent (As^{+3}), pentavalent (As^{+5})
- Range of toxicity: arsine > trivalent > pentavalent > elemental[1]
- Organic arsenic may be present in seafood, is nontoxic, and is cleared within days from the body.
- Arsenic is well absorbed via GI or respiratory routes and distributed to all body tissues.
- Arsenic impairs cellular respiration, inhibits sulfhydryl-containing enzymes, and may substitute for phosphates in high-energy compounds.[10,11]
- Cancers associated with arsenic
  - Lung, bladder, skin leukemia, lymphoma

Lead

- Major route of exposure is ingestion or inhalation.
- Most of lead in bloodstream is bound to red blood cells, but lead is also stored in soft tissue and bone.

- Binds to sulfhydryl groups and other proteins, causes abnormal hemoglobin synthesis, and interferes with numerous metabolic processes
- Lead is structurally similar to calcium and interferes with calcium-mediated processes.
- Children absorb 40% to 50% of ingested lead; adults absorb 10% to 15%.[2]

Mercury

- Multiple forms: elemental, inorganic, organic
- Elemental mercury is a mobile, liquid metal, and exposure is typically through inhalation. Elemental Hg is poorly absorbed in the GI tract.
- Inorganic mercury is primarily absorbed via the GI tract and is corrosive.
- Mercury is a general protoplasmic poison and binds to sulfhydryl groups.
- Organic mercury or methylmercury is found in seafood and shellfish and primarily absorbed via the GI tract.

Metal Fume Fever

- Caused by exposure to metal oxide fumes, which are small particles formed by vaporization of metals with subsequent condensation.[8]
- Its pathogenesis is poorly understood, but metal oxide fumes may have direct toxic effects on the respiratory tract or may cause a delayed hypersensitivity reaction.[15]

Clinical Presentations

Arsenic

- Diagnosis is based on appropriate symptoms and elevated urine arsenic levels.
- Acute arsenic ingestion may cause acute nausea, vomiting, abdominal pain, or diarrhea within minutes to hours of exposure.[1,12]
- Arsenic toxicity may cause cardiovascular instability, hypotension, intravascular volume depletion, myocardial dysfunction, a **prolonged QT interval,** and dysrrthymia.[10,12]
- Severe poisoning may result in coma, acute encephalopathy, fevers, pulmonary edema, respiratory failure, toxic hepatitis, rhabdomyolysis, acute renal failure, GI ulcerative lesions, hemorrhage, seizures, and death.[1,2]

- Subacute or long-term symptoms may include anemia, leukopenia, aplastic anemia, or sensory motor neuropathy (more sensory symptoms than motor).
- *Subcute or chronic skin findings include:* hyperkeratosis of palms and soles, alopecia, keratosis, desquamation, pigmentation changes, and eczematous changes.[2,10]
- Arsenic exposure has been linked to lung cancer, skin cancer, and bladder cancer.
- Arsine gas is a colorless, nonirritating gas and causes triad of abdominal pain, hematuria, and jaundice due to massive hemolysis.

Lead

- May cause multisystem signs and symptoms including:
  - With acute lead poisoning, GI symptoms such as anorexia, abdominal pain (lead colic), constipation, and vomiting
  - Normochromic or microcytic anemia (with basophilic stippling)
  - Neurologic symptoms such as headache, fatigue, irritability, tremor, encephalopathy, and coma
- Overt encephalopathy is more common in children with a BLL over 100 µg/dL but may occur with BBLs as low as 70 µg/dL.[2]
- Adults with overt encephalopathy typically have BLLs >100 µg/dL.[3]
- Lead poisoning may also cause a peripheral neuropathy (**more motor than sensory**), vague aches and pains, and renal disease.
- Reproductive effects include infertility, stillbirth, cognitive dysfunction in children, spontaneous abortions, and decreased sperm counts.[2,3]
- Children have more symptoms than adults at comparable BLLs.

Mercury

- Diagnosis of mercury toxicity is based on appropriate symptoms following an exposure.
- Elemental mercury
  - Elemental mercury may cause cough, chills, fever, metal fume fever, interstitial pneumonitis, and fibrosis.[6,10]
  - See Boxes 12-5 and 12-6.
  - Erethism symptoms include shyness, anxiety, emotional lability, irritability (think Mad Hatter), delirium, and Parkinson disease-like features.[7]

- Ingestion of elemental mercury (liquid at room temperature) is relatively harmless unless the mercury becomes trapped in the gut.[10]
- Inorganic mercury salts such as in mercury disc battery[7] (Box 12-7)
- **Ingestion of organic or alkyl mercury** (Box 12-8)

Box 12-5 ▪ POSSIBLE RESULTS OF CHRONIC EXPOSURE TO MERCURY	
Tremors	Gingivitis
Cheilitis	Rash
Erethism	Fatigue
Headaches	Stomatitis

Box 12-6 ▪ CLINICAL EFFECTS OF ELEMENTAL MERCURY INHALATION
Cough, chills, shortness of breath, fever
Metallic taste, nausea, vomiting, diarrhea, headache
Interstitial pneumonitis

Box 12-7 ▪ CLINICAL EFFECTS OF INORGANIC MERCURY SALTS	
Irritant or caustic gastrointestinal irritation	Bloody diarrhea
Acute renal failure	Circulatory collapse
Tremor	Erethism

Box 12-8 ▪ ORGANIC MERCURY
CNS symptoms
Paresthesias
Tremor
Ataxia
Dysarthria
Dementia
Tunnel vision
Maternal exposure
Cerebral palsy-type abnormalities
Mental retardation
Seizures
Cataracts
Hearing loss
CNS abnormalities (in the fetus)

- Mercury may also cause allergic contact dermatitis or urticaria.

Metal Fume Fever

- Metal fume fever results in flulike symptoms.
- Complete recovery usually occurs within 24–48 hr, with no permanent lung damage.
- Patients typically present within 3–12 hr of exposure (median 5 hr).[8]
- See Box 12-9.
- Most of the patients have a fever on presentation (90% are febrile).
- Chest radiographs are usually normal but may show a diffuse increase in bronchovascular markings.

Laboratory Evaluation

Arsenic

- Normal whole blood arsenic is <5 µg/L, and normal 24-hr urine arsenic is <50 µg/L, with an action level for urine >100 µg/L.[1]
- Urine arsenic levels are more useful and reliable than blood levels.
- Organic arsenic from seafood or shellfish ingestion
  - May cause an elevated urine arsenic level for several days, up to 2000 µg/L[10]
  - Is relatively nontoxic and is rapidly cleared from the body. Therefore it is important to speciate the total arsenic level (determine whether it is organic or inorganic, trivalent, or pentavalent).[13,14]
- Hair and nail arsenic may be reliable for long-term exposure.[12]
- *Consider ordering the following tests in the ED:*
  - CBC, electrolytes, BUN/Cr

Box 12-9 ■ Metal Fume Fever Presentation	
Fever	Chills
Headache	Myalgia, cough
Shortness of breath*	Metallic taste in mouth*
Nausea and vomiting*	Rales on exam

Complaints in some patients.

- ECG
- Arsenic level (preferably 24-hr urine, although spot urine may be used in emergency) with speciations (it may be a few days before you receive results in most EDs)
- Consider abdominal and chest radiographs (looking for radiopaque material) if acute ingestion.

Lead

- Whole blood lead is the best screening tool for lead toxicity. A normal BLL is <10 µg/dL.[2]
- Always confirm an elevated capillary or fingerstick BLL with a venous or whole BLL.
- BLL may be an unreliable indicator of whole body lead burden or bone lead levels in those with chronic or remote poisoning.
- Erythrocyte protoporphyrin is not sufficiently sensitive for screening but may reflect chronic toxicity.[15]
- In lead-poisoned children, lead lines may be seen on radiographs of long bones.
- X-ray fluorescence is available in some parts of the country and can be used to document lead body burden.
- *Order the following tests in the ED:*
  - CBC with differential, BUN, Cr
  - BLL
  - Abdominal radiograph
  - Rule out other etiology for patient's symptoms because BLL results will probably **not** be received quickly.

Mercury

- Normal whole blood mercury level is <10 µg/dL, but the action level is greater than 35 µg/dL. Normal 24-hr urine mercury level is <20 µg/dL, and the action level is >150 µg/dL.[16]
- Urine mercury may correlate with inorganic mercury toxicity but is not as useful for methylmercury or organic mercury toxicity (for methylmercury or organic mercury, use blood mercury instead).
- Elevated urine or blood mercury levels may occur after seafood or fish consumption.
- *Order the following tests in the ED:*
  - Electrolytes, BUN, Cr
  - Urinalysis
  - 24-hour urine mercury, blood mercury
  - Consider abdominal x-ray if recent ingestion.[10]

Metal Fume Fever

- There is no pathognomic laboratory test for metal fume fever.
- A history of classic symptoms after exposure to metal fumes in the workplace, particularly in operations involving heating of metals shown to cause metal fume fever, is the key to diagnosis.[9]
- A chest x-ray should be ordered to evaluate for pneumonitis.

■ Treatment

Arsenic

- Requires good supportive care.
- If radiopaque material is present in the GI tract, then lavage or activated charcoal followed by whole bowel irrigation is appropriate.
- Avoid medication that will prolong the QT interval.
- A severely ill patient in whom arsenic poisoning is suspected may be started on chelation prior to your receipt of urine arsenic results.
- Severe arsenic toxicity with significant GI and CNS symptoms plus elevated blood or urine arsenic levels is usually treated by British anti-lewisite (BAL): 3–5 mg/kg IM every 4–6 hr until the 24-hr urine is <50 µg/L or 2,3-dimercaptosuccinic acid (DMSA).[2] DMSA appears more effective than BAL (BAL may increase brain arsenic levels) but has not been approved by the FDA for arsenic toxicity.[10]
- DMSA is well tolerated and may be the chelator of choice for subacute or chronic toxicity.
  - **Dose:** DMSA 10 mg/kg tid for 5 days, then 10 mg/kg for 14 days[10,11]

Lead

- It is important to evaluate the source of the lead exposure in every patient with an elevated BLL to determine whether significant exposure has occurred.
- Treatment is based on BLL, age of the patient, and severity of symptoms.
- If radiopaque material is present in the GI tract, then lavage followed by whole bowel irrigation is appropriate.

- DMSA is the chelator of choice in the United States unless the patient presents with protracted vomiting, severe toxicity, or encephalopathy (usually a child).[15]
- Patients with overt encephalopathy are treated with:
  - BAL ($75 \, mg/m^2$ IM every 4 hr for 5 days) plus
  - $CaNa_2$ EDTA started 4 hr after the BAL at a dose of $1500 \, mg/m^2$ per day as a continuous infusion or in 2–4 divided IV doses for 3–5 days[2]
- Symptomatic adults with BLL >100 μg/dL or symptomatic children or any child with BLL >70 μg/dL are treated with:
  - BAL ($50–75 \, mg/m^2$ IM q 4 hr for 5 days) plus
  - $CaNa_2$ EDTA started 4 hr after the BAL at a dose of $1000–1500 \, mg/m^2$ per day as a continuous infusion or in 2–4 divided IV doses for 3–5 days[2]
- Symptomatic adults or symptomatic children or asymptomatic children with BLL >45 μg/dL may be treated with:
  - Oral DMSA or succimer given as 10 mg/kg or 350 mg/m^2 tid for 5 days, then bid for 14 days[2]
- Chelation may not be indicated in asymptomatic adults with BLL <70 μg/dL, but they should be removed from lead exposure[2] and followed with serial BLLs. Draw repeat BLL several days after each course of chelation, and if it is still elevated, a repeat course of treatment may be recommended.

Mercury

- General supportive care is appropriate treatment.
- Elemental inhalation: Monitor respiratory status.
- If an inorganic salt was ingested and corrosive lesions or ulcers are concerns, then GI upper endoscopy should be considered before lavage and whole bowel irrigation are performed.
- If metallic mercury is seen in the GI tract on the abdominal radiograph, then activated charcoal followed by whole bowel irritation is appropriate.
- Oral DMSA is the preferred chelator if the patient has normal renal function.[7]
- BAL may be contraindicated with methylmercury.[10]
- DMSA is given as 10 mg/kg tid for 5 days, then bid for 14 days.[12]
- Chelation with BAL is appropriate if there is renal dysfunction or severe toxicity.[7]

Metal Fume Fever

- General supportive care such as use of oxygen, IV fluids, and antipyretics is appropriate.
- Antacids may alleviate GI symptoms such as nausea and vomiting.
- Glucocorticoids have been used in patients with severe symptoms or interstitial infiltrates, but their efficacy has not been well proven.
- Preventing or minimizing subsequent exposure is essential.
- Recommending good worksite ventilation is important; respiratory protection may also be needed.
- Cadmium inhalation may cause more severe pneumonitis.[15]

Special Considerations

Arsenic

Arsenic-contaminated drinking water is present in numerous areas around the world, but in many areas results in low-level exposure.

Lead

- Children are more sensitive to adverse effects of lead.
- Children absorb 40%–50% of ingested lead; adults absorb only 10%–15%.
- Children tend to be more symptomatic than adults at a given BLL and are more susceptible to CNS toxicity than adults.
- In pregnancy:
  - Lead crosses the placental barrier and is found in breast milk.
  - Elevated lead levels may cause infertility, low birth weight, cognitive dysfunction in child, and spontaneous abortions.
  - Remove pregnant woman with elevated BLL from exposure and consider chelating the pregnant woman with severe lead toxicity. However, there is a theoretical risk of teratogenesis or fetal effect in early pregnancy.[2]

Mercury

- FDA recommendations for women who might become pregnant, pregnant woman, nursing mothers, and young children:

- Do not eat shark, swordfish, king mackerel, or tilefish.
- Eat up to 12 oz (2 average meals) per week of a variety of fish and shellfish that are lower in mercury (e.g., shrimp, canned light tuna, salmon, pollock, catfish).
- Check local advisories about the safety of fish caught by family or friends.[5]

Admission Criteria

Arsenic

- Severe toxicity, cardiac toxicity
- Psychiatric evaluation if suicidal

Lead

Encephalopathy, severe CNS toxicity, severe vomiting

Mercury

Life-threatening toxicity, renal failure, acute pneumonitis with respiratory distress[7]

Metal Fume Fever

Moderate or severe respiratory distress and pneumonitis; observe for 24 to 48 hr.

Pearls and Pitfalls

- If a patient has arsenic, mercury, or lead toxicity, then it is important to evaluate the source of the exposure and remove or minimize future exposures.
- Check renal function and urine output before giving BAL or DMSA because both increase urinary excretion of metals.
- Lead, arsenic, and mercury all cause GI, renal, and neurologic symptoms.
- Urine arsenic is more reliable than blood arsenic.
- Blood lead is more reliable than urine lead.
- Venous blood is more specific for lead poisoning and more reliable than capillary blood.[15]
- Blood mercury is more reliable for organic or methylmercury exposure.

- The CDC recommends clinical intervention if a child's BLL is >10 µg/dL.
- Children are more likely than adults to become symptomatic from lead toxicity.

References and Suggested Reading

1. Yip L, Dart RC: Arsenic. In Sullivan J, Krieger G, eds: *Clinical environmental health and toxic exposures*, ed 2, Philadelphia, 2001, Lippincott, Williams & Wilkins, pp 858–866.

2. Henretig FM: Lead. In Goldfrank LR, Flomenbaum NE, Lewin NA, et al, eds: *Goldfrank's toxicologic emergencies*, ed 7, New York, 2002, McGraw-Hill, pp 1200–1227.

3. Kosnett MJ: Lead. In Ford MD, Delaney KA, Ling LJ, et al, eds: *Clinical toxicology*, Philadelphia, 2001, WB Saunders, pp 723–736.

4. Keogh JP, Boyer LV: Lead. In Sullivan J, Krieger G, eds: *Clinical environmental health and toxic exposures*, ed 2, Philadelphia, 2001, Lippincott, Williams & Wilkins, pp 879–888.

5. United States Environmental Protection Agency, US DHHS: *What you need to know about mercury in fish and shellfish*, March 2004: www.cfsan.fda.gov.

6. Yip L, Dart RC, Sullivan JB: Mercury. In Sullivan J, Krieger G, eds: *Hazardous material toxicology: clinical principles of environmental health*, Baltimore, 2002, Williams & Wilkins, pp 867–878.

7. Chiang WK: Mercury. In Ford MD, Delaney KA, Ling LJ, et al, eds: *Clinical toxicology*, Philadelphia, 2001, WB Saunders, pp 737–743.

8. Baker BA: Metal fume fever. In Ford MD, Delaney KA, Ling LJ, et al, eds: *Clinical toxicology*, Philadelphia, 2001, WB Saunders, pp 699–704.

9. Farrell FJ: Metal oxides. In Sullivan J, Krieger G, eds: *Clinical environmental health and toxic exposures*, ed 2, Philadelphia, 2001, Lippincott, Williams & Wilkins, pp 973–977.

10. Graeme KA, Pollack CV Jr: Heavy metal toxicity. Part I: arsenic and mercury, *J Emerg Med* 16:45–56, 1998.

11. Ford MD: Arsenic. In Goldfrank LR, Flomenbaum NE, Lewin NA, et al, eds: *Goldfrank's toxicologic emergencies*, ed 7, New York, 2002, McGraw-Hill, pp 1183–1195.

12. Hryhorczuk D, Eng J: Arsenic in clinical toxicology. In Ford MD, Delaney KA, Ling LJ, et al, eds: *Clinical toxicology*, Philadelphia, 2001, WB Saunders, pp 716–721.

13. Farmer JD, Johnson LR: Assessment of occupational exposure of inorganic arsenic based on urinary concentrations and speciation of arsenic, *Br J Industr Med* 47:342–348, 1990.

14. Halaka, E, Pyy L: Assessment of exposure to inorganic arsenic by determining the arsenic species excreted in urine, *Toxicol Ltrs* 77:249–258, 1995.

15. Graeme KA, Pollack CJ: Heavy metal toxicity. Part II: lead and metal fume fever, *J Emerg Med* 16:171–177, 1998.

16. Sue YJ: Mercury. In Goldfrank LR, Flomenbaum NE, Lewin NA, et al, eds: *Goldfrank's toxicologic emergencies*, ed 7, New York, 2002, McGraw-Hill, pp 1239–1248.

Chapter 13

Caustic Ingestions

PETER KUMASAKA

Overview

Caustics damage tissue through chemical reactions, which cause thermal reactions, alter chemical bonds, and denature proteins. A caustic's strength is determined by the pH (or pKa) of the acid-base. Generally, pH levels <2 (strong acid) or >12 (strong base) produce the worst injuries. Other characteristics affect the injury severity. These include the volume of neutralizing agent needed to bring pH to a normal physiologic level (the titratable acid/alkali reserve [TAR]), the concentration, duration of contact, volume of the caustic, volume and contents of the stomach, and the ability of the caustic to penetrate the tissue.

Substances

Many caustics can be found both in the home and at work. Generally, caustics used in the industrial or occupational setting are more highly concentrated. As a result, on-the-job caustic exposures are potentially more toxic and injurious.

Alkaline Substances

Sodium hydroxide	Calcium carbide	Caustic soda
Sodium carbonate	Caustic potash	Sodium silicate
Sodium hypochlorite	Potassium carbonate	Potassium hydroxide
Ammonia	Sodium metasilicate	Potassium metasilicate
Lime	Sodium oxide	Calcium oxide
Sodium phosphate	Trisodium phosphate	Lye

Alkaline Products

Bleach, household (4%–6% Na hypochlorite)	Dishwasher detergent
Oven cleaners	Alkaline batteries
Drain cleaners	Mildew removers
Toilet bowl cleaners	Hair care products, dyes
Glass cleaners	Cement (calcium oxide)
Clinitest tabs (sodium hydroxide, sodium carbonate)	Desiccants packets (outside the U.S.)

Acid Substances and Uses

Products	Substances
Sulfuric acid	Toilet bowl and drain cleaners, automobile batteries, fertilizers
Hydrochloric acid	Metal cleaners, toilet bowl cleaners, bleaching agents
Phosphoric acid	Rust removers, disinfectants
Hydrofluoric acid	Disinfects, antirust solutions
Nitric acid	Engraving solutions
Oxalic acid	Blueprint paper, tanning
Acetic acid	Hair-wave neutralizers
Citric acid	Diluting agent and food preservative

■ Toxicity

- See Box 13-1.
- Systemic acidosis may also occur from direct absorption of large acid ingestion, shock and hemolysis, and/or tissue necrosis with lactate production.

BOX 13-1 ▪ ACID/BASE INJURY PATTERNS	
A*c*ids	A*L*kali
Coagulative necrosis	**Liquefactive necrosis**
Eschar formation: limits penetration Exception: hydrofluoric acid	Initial injury occurs nearly instantaneously Saponifies and can continue to penetrate Oropharynx/esophagus more commonly involved than stomach
Acute injury	**Acute injury**
Primarily gastric injury 6%–20% esophageal Rare to have acute perforation	Burn Edema and airway obstruction Perforation of esophagus or stomach can occur early
Delayed or late	**Delayed or late**
Perforation can occur when eschar sloughs in 3–4 days Outlet obstruction	Stricture formation Fistula Cancer (squamous cell cancer of esophagus) Fibrosis of posterior cricoarytenoid muscles

- Caustic injuries greatly increase the risk of squamous cell cancer of the esophagus (1000× that of the general population).
- Mean onset of cancer after caustic exposure is 45 years.

Clinical Presentation

- See Table 13-1.
- Minimal physical findings may **not** be a reliable indicator of severity.
- Patients can be symptomatic without significant injury.
- See Box 13-2.
- High anion gap or nonanion gap metabolic acidosis may be present.

Diagnostic Testing

- CBC, electrolytes including Mg, P, Ca
- Coagulation studies

Table 13-1 INJURY SEVERITY AND COMPLICATIONS

Grade	Findings	Comments
Grade 0	No injury	No adverse effects
Grade I	Erythema, edema	No adverse sequelae
Grade II	limited to mucosa	
Grade IIb (circumferential)	Blister, ulcerations, and whitish membrane penetrating the mucosa	Grade IIb may develop strictures
Grade III	Extensive necrosis, full thickness or frank perforation	High morbidity and mortality May result in perforation, mediastinitis, or peritonitis Strictures seen in majority

---

BOX 13-2 ▪ PRESENTATION AND FINDINGS

Dysphagia	Oropharyngeal pain or swelling
Chest pain	Abdominal pain
Stridor	Hoarseness
Peritonitis	Hypotension
Hematemesis	

Systemic problems

Renal failure	Electrolyte disturbance
Metabolic acidosis	Hemolysis

- pH of substance
- Blood pH may be useful to determine the extent of injury.

Imaging

- Chest radiograph and abdominal series
    - Generally only useful in the acute stage of management if positive findings are present
        - Pneumomediastinum
        - Free air
        - Pleural effusion/infiltrates (aspiration pneumonia)
        - Viscus perforation
    - Negative findings do not exclude GI tract perforation.
- Contrast studies
    - Used when there is a suspicion of perforation, and distal esophagus is not seen (because of proximal esophageal injury or circumferential burns).
    - Serial studies may be useful.

- Dye extravasation is diagnostic but may not locate all perforations.
- Signs of significant necrosis and impending perforation
- Dilatation of the esophagus
- Pleural reflection displacement
- Widening of the pleuroesophageal line
- CT scan has not been studied sufficiently in caustic ingestions to offer reliable guidance in management.

Treatment

- ABCs and supportive care
  - Airway: Avoid paralytics and blind intubation. Fiberoptics may be required.
  - IV line
  - ECG monitor if hydrofluoric acid
- Decontamination
  - Copious lavage with water for skin and eyes
  - Gastric lavage only in serious, large **acid** ingestion
    - Use small NG tube due to the risk of perforation.
  - **NO activated charcoal and NO emetics**
  - Emesis leads to reexposure to caustics.
    - Risk of aspiration
  - Charcoal does not bind most agents.
    - Obscures view for EGD
    - Risk of emesis
- Dilution
  - Consider **dilutional** therapy (H_2O) if **<30 min** post-ingestion and **NOT** a strong acid.
  - Wash out any crystals or adherent material in the mouth.
  - H_2O or milk (small amount)
  - **Remember: In order to change the pH by 1 point, you need to dilute the solution tenfold.**
  - Consider the possibility of an exothermic reaction causing further tissue injury.
- Obtain any information regarding the caustic agent.

Substances

Acid or base (alkali)?	How much?
Concentration?	Coingestants?
When taken?	Solid or liquid?

- Consider NG/OG, if **early**, to remove excess liquid, although there are no clear clinical trials to support this.
  - **NOT** if known alkali or unknown ingestion
- **Consult** for urgent **EGD**
  - Within 12 hr postingestion
  - Controversial whether asymptomatic patients need to be scoped
  - Some studies suggest that asymptomatic children do not need EGD.
- Steroids
  - Currently, **no study indicates the effectiveness of steroids** to improve outcome.
  - Some animal studies show lower stricture formation.
  - A few human studies show improvement but also higher acute morbidity and mortality.
  - Use in consultation with GI or surgical consultant.
    - May be useful in Grade II injuries
    - Initiate within 48 hr of injury.
    - Dose recommendations:
      - 20 mg methylprednisolone Q 8 hr if <2 yrs old
      - 40 mg methylprednisolone Q 8 hr if >2 yrs old
      - Oral regimen is prednisone 2 mg/kg QD × 2–3 weeks, then 1-month taper.
- Antibiotics
  - No indication that prophylactic antibiotics help reduce morbidity or mortality
  - Use in conjunction with steroids or if evidence of infection and/or perforation.
    - Oral flora and anaerobes coverage (i.e., clindamycin)
- Surgery
  - If evidence of perforation
  - No good criteria for early surgical intervention

Special Considerations

Hydrofluoric Acid (HF)

- Used mostly in glass etching, but also in rust removers, graffiti removal, wheel cleaners, and jewelry work
- Very caustic and acts more like a base (**liquefactive** necrosis)
- Most issues related to dermal exposure
  - Could lead to hypocalcemia, so check calcium, magnesium, and potassium levels.
  - Treatment: calcium gluconate

- Topical
  - Apply 2.5% calcium gluconate gel to the affected area.
  - The pharmacy can make this by dissolving 10% calcium gluconate solution in 3× the volume of KY Gel (water-soluble lubricant).
- Intradermal
  - Not recommended due to risk of tissue damage; it causes severe pain.
- IV
- Dilute 10–15 mL of 10% calcium gluconate plus 5000 U heparin with up to 40 ml D_5W.
- Use Bier block to infuse, but release the cuff if any of the following occur:
  - Pain resolves.
  - Cuff becomes more painful than the burn.
  - Cuff has been inflated for +20 minutes.
- May repeat in 4 hr prn
- Continuous ECG monitoring is essential.
- Intra-arterial
  - An A-line (arterial catheter) in the radial or brachial artery. **Be sure that** the catheter is in the artery, by using continuous waveform analysis. Avoid the risk of tissue necrosis and digit loss from extravasation of calcium (remember, do no harm).
  - Infuse a solution of 10 mL of 10% calcium gluconate in 40 mL of D_5W over a 4-hr period.
  - May need to repeat several times after 4- to 8-hr interval from end of last treatment
  - Continuous ECG and clinical monitoring are essential.
- Ingestion
  - Once systemic, will bind up calcium and cause **severe hypocalcemia.**
  - Can lead to rapid deterioration, dysrhythmias, and death.

Oxalic Acid

- Mild corrosive
- Binds calcium, causing hypocalcemia
- Precipitates can cause renal damage.

Zinc and Mercuric Chloride

- Same supportive care for other corrosives
- Risk of heavy metal poisoning

- Activated charcoal may be useful. There is some evidence that it can adsorb some of these agents.
  - Gentle NG lavage
- May need chelation therapy

Admission Criteria

- Evidence of perforation
- Any airway involvement
- Extensive alkali burns
- Severe pain
- EKG changes
- Inability to tolerate PO
- Intentional ingestion
- Toxic coingestants

Pearls and Pitfalls

- Have a high level of suspicion for worse problems, despite minimal symptoms.
- Absence of oropharyngeal burns does not rule out significant visceral injury.
- Do not neutralize.
- Consider dilutional therapy only in limited cases.
- Consult GI early for EGD (within 12–24 hrs).
- Suicidal patients tend to minimize symptoms. Their history and physical exam are unreliable, so early endoscopy is required (6–12 hr postingestion).
- For HF exposures to fingertips, calcium gluconate gel may be placed in an exam glove for the patient to wear.

Suggested Readings

1. Anderson KD, Rouse TM, Randolph JG: A controlled trial of corticosteroids in children with corrosive injury of the esophagus, *N Engl J Med* 323:637–640, 1990.
2. Ellenhorn MJ, Schonwald S, Ordug G, Wasserberger J, eds: Household poisonings. In *Ellenhorn's medical toxicology*, ed 2, Baltimore, 1997, Williams & Wilkins, pp 1078–1097.
3. Gupta SK, Croffie JM, Fitzgerald JF: Is esophagogastroduodenoscopy necessary in all caustic ingestions? *J Pediatr Gastroenterol Nutr* 32:8–10, 2001.
4. Kardon E: Toxicity, caustic ingestions. In Kreplick LW, Van De Voort JT, Burns MJ, et al., eds: *eMedicine* (online). *eMedicine J*, May 9, 2001.
5. Lamireau T, Rebouissoux L, Denis D, et al: Accidental caustic ingestion in children: is endoscopy always mandatory? *J Pediatr Gastroenterol Nutr* 33:81–84, 2001.

6. Rao RB, Hoffman RS: Caustics and batteries. In Goldfrank LR, Flomenbaum NE, Lewin NA, et al, eds: *Goldfrank's toxicologic emergencies*, ed 7, New York, 2002, McGraw-Hill, pp 1323–1340.

7. Schaffer SB, Hebert AF: Caustic ingestion, *J La State Med Soc* 152:590–596, 2000.

8. Ulman I, Mutaf O: A critique of systemic steroids in the management of caustic esophageal burns in children, *Eur J Pediatr Surg* 8:71–74, 1998.

Chapter 14

Hydrocarbons

Brad Hernandez

Overview

Hydrocarbons (HCs) are organic compounds made of primarily carbon and hydrogen molecules. The majority are liquid products of petroleum or wood distillation whose toxicity is directly related to their physical properties and the presence of any side chains. In general, a lower viscosity, higher volatility, and lower surface tension lead to an increased risk of injury.

The American Association of Poison Control Centers estimates there are 60,000 HC exposures annually. Approximately 95% are unintentional; 60% involve children; approximately 20 exposures annually are fatal; and 90% of fatalities are children. Siphoning and inhalant abuse cause a significant number of exposures. The volatilized substance is absorbed from the respiratory system within seconds and is quickly distributed to the CNS. The most commonly abused substances are paints, varnishes, glues, gasoline, lighter fluids, and aerosol propellants.

▌Substances

Classification			
Aliphatics (Straight or Branched Chain)	**Cyclic Hydrocarbon (Closed Ring)**		
	Aromatics	**Alicyclics**	**Cyclic Terpenes**
Paraffins	Benzenes - 1 ring	Cycloparaffins - naphthenes	Essential oils (plant origin)
Olefins - Alkenes (double bonds) - Alkadienes (2 double bonds) - Acetylenes (triple bond) Acyclic terpenes	Naphthalenes - 2 rings Anthracenes - 3 rings Polycyclic Heterocyclic	Cycloolefins - (2 or more double bonds)	

Hydrocarbon Exposures	
Gasoline (most common)	Freon
Mineral spirits	Motor oils
Lighter fluids	Kerosene

Household products

Adhesives	Baby oil
Car wax	Contact cement
Furniture polish	Lacquers
Mineral spirits	Mothballs
Lamp oils	Paint removers and thinners
Paraffin	Petroleum jelly
Pine oils	Solvents
Stain removers	Turpentine
Typewriter correction fluid	

Commonly Inhaled Substances of Abuse	
Paints	Varnishes
Glues	Gasoline
Lighter fluids	Aerosol propellants (air fresheners)

◼ Toxicity

- The primary organ system affected is the pulmonary system.
  - HCs induce aspiration, resulting in direct toxicity to pulmonary tissue.
  - Interstitial inflammation
  - Polymorphonuclear leukocyte (PMN) exudation
  - Intraalveolar hemorrhage and edema
  - Hyperemic blood vessels
  - Bronchial necrosis
  - Vascular thrombosis
  - Impairment of the lipid surfactant layer
- Halogenated HCs cause CNS depression and possibly hepatotoxicity
  - Worst hepatotoxicity: Carbon tetrachloride (CCl_4) and trichloromethane (chloroform)
  - Intermediate toxicity: tetrachloroethane and trichloroethylene
  - Weakest hepatotoxicity: tetrachloroethylene, trichloroethane, and dichloromethane
  - Renal toxicity parallels hepatotoxicity.
- Inhaled aromatic and short-chain HCs have a rapid, intoxicating effect.
  - The volatilized substance is absorbed from the respiratory system within seconds and quickly distributed to the CNS.
  - Myocardial sensitization to catecholamines
  - May lead to "sudden sniffing death"

◼ Clinical Presentation

- Most patients will have immediate choking or gagging. Pulmonary toxicity develops within hours with rales, bronchospasm, hypoxia, hemoptysis, pulmonary edema, or respiratory distress.
- Other organ systems affected include CNS, GI, cardiac, and skin. The CNS effects are coma and seizures, presumptively from pulmonary absorption and hypoxia or direct toxic properties.
- GI complaints are generally mild; however, vomiting is common and may increase the risk of pulmonary toxicity.
- There is also risk of dysrhythmias and sudden death after large exposures, especially in cases of intentional abuse.
- Acute prolonged exposures can cause severe, full-thickness skin burns.

- Radiographic evidence of pneumonitis develops between 15 min and 24 hr postingestion.
  - 90% of patients develop radiographic changes within 4 hr of ingestion.
  - Most patients who have respiratory symptoms in excess of gagging and choking will go on to develop radiographic changes.
  - Common radiologic findings include bronchovascular markings, bibasilar infiltrates, and consolidation.
  - Right-sided and lower lobe lung involvement are more common.
- Respiratory failure is frequently due to a ventilation/perfusion mismatch. Positive end-expiratory pressure (PEEP) is helpful. In most significant exposures, respiratory symptoms improve in 72 hr with standard respiratory therapy.

Laboratory Evaluation

- ABG to assess degree of hypoxemia
  - Hypercarbia may be present.
- Basic metabolic panel to assess presence of increased anion gap and possible coingestion of another agent
- Imaging
  - Chest radiography in all symptomatic patients
  - Common findings include atelectasis, fine perihilar opacities, and bibasilar infiltrates.
  - Pneumothorax or pneumomediastinum may develop.
- Other tests
  - Bedside pulse oximetry to assess for hypoxia due to HC aspiration
- ECG

Treatment

- ABCs, supplemental oxygen, IV, and cardiac monitor
- If obtunded, consider naloxone, dextrose, and thiamine.
- If clothing is involved, it should be removed.
  - Caregivers should be cautious to avoid self-contamination.
- Decontamination
  - Gastric emptying is rarely indicated because gastrointestinal absorption is minimal.
  - If the patient is asymptomatic, observe without decontamination.

- Gastric lavage is generally considered the procedure of choice for large, intentional overdoses (i.e., greater than 30 ml) or other toxic coingestions.
- In addition, CHAMP substances all warrant gastric emptying due to their inherent systemic toxicity and potential for delayed toxic effects:
    - **C**amphor
    - **H**alogenated HCs
    - **A**romatic HCs
    - **M**etal-associated HCs
    - **P**esticide-associated HCs
- If no other ingested substance is suspected, an 18F NG tube is sufficient for lavage with airway protection if there is loss of gag reflex.
- Ipecac-induced emesis is contraindicated due to the risk and severity of potential aspiration.
- Dermal exposures require clothing removal, copious irrigation, and soap cleansing.
- For the treatment of pulmonary symptoms, corticosteroids are contraindicated and antibiotics are controversial.
    - Some authors recommend that severely poisoned patients receive antibiotics to prevent bacterial superinfection.
- Respiratory failure is frequently due to a ventilation/perfusion mismatch. PEEP is helpful. In most significant exposures, respiratory symptoms improve in 72 hr with standard respiratory therapy.
- Because free radical formation initiates lipid peroxidation and subsequent hepatic necrosis, *N*-acetylcysteine (NAC) is advocated by some authors in significant carbon tetrachloride exposures.

Special Considerations

- Prolonged exposure or heated HC can cause full-thickness burns.
    - Tar and asphalt are hot HCs that cause severe burns on exposed skin. Immediate cooling with cold water is followed by complete removal. HC ointment (De-Solv-it, Tween-80, Polysorbate 80) is combined with a surface agent (Neosporin or petroleum jelly).
    - There is also potential for inhalation injury from toxic gases.
- High-pressure injection gun injuries cause significant destruction and require emergent surgical debridement.

- Volatile substance abuse
  - The toxic effects are primarily cardiac and neurologic.
  - CNS effects are stupor, excitation, agitation, hallucinations, seizures, ataxia, headache, and dizziness.
  - Cardiac effects are potentially fatal dysrhythmias and sudden death ("sudden sniffing death").
    - This most commonly occurs when abuse is followed with an adrenaline rush such as running, fear, or sexual activity.
    - Epinephrine is not recommended as a first-line agent in ventricular tachycardia or fibrillation.
    - Treatment in a nonfatal exposure includes keeping the patient in a dark, quiet room with minimal stimulation.

Admission Criteria

- The majority of patients exposed to HC do not need to be admitted.
- If discharge is being considered for an asymptomatic patient, a chest radiograph should be obtained 6 hr postingestion to document the negative findings.
- Patients with no initial symptoms and no hypoxia, respiratory distress, nor radiographic evidence of pneumonitis after 6 hr of observation can be safely discharged.
- Intentional ingestions and CHAMP substances require admission.

Pearls and Pitfalls

- HCs can be "huffed," "sniffed," or "bagged."
  - *Huffing* refers to pouring hydrocarbon onto a sock or rag, *sniffing* is usually pouring it into a container, and *bagging* is inhalation from a paper or plastic bag.
- *N*-acetylcysteine (NAC) is advocated by some authors in significant carbon tetrachloride exposures.
- Oral frostbite can occur from attempts to inhale freon or fluorinated HCs.

References and Suggested Readings

1. Anas N, Namasonthi V, Ginsburg CM: Criteria for hospitalizing children who have ingested products containing hydrocarbons, *JAMA* 246:840-843, 1981.

2. Anene O, Castello FV: Myocardial dysfunction after hydrocarbon ingestion, *Crit Care Med* 22:528-530, 1994.

3. Dice WH, Ward G, Kelley J, et al: Pulmonary toxicity following gastrointestinal ingestion of kerosene, *Ann Emerg Med* 11:138-142, 1982 [canine study].

4. Goldstein RJ, Haynes JF Jr: Toxicity, hydrocarbons. *eMedicine*. Last Updated: October 26, 2004.

5. Henretig FM: Special considerations in the poisoned pediatric patient, *Emerg Med Clin North Am* 12:549-567, 1994.

6. MacFarland HN: Toxicology of solvents, *Am Indust Hyg Assoc J* 47:704-707, 1986.

7. Von Oettingen WF: Toxicity and potential dangers of aliphatic and aromatic hydrocarbons. A critical review of the literature, *U.S. Public Health Bulletin* 255, 1940.

Chapter 15

Toxic Gases

Brad Hernandez

1. Cyanide

Overview

Hydrogen cyanide (HCN) toxicity occurs by inhalation, ingestion, and cutaneous and parenteral exposures. It is available in chemical laboratories and used in electroplating, metal refining, photography, jewelry cleaner, fertilizers, and fumigation. It may be used as chemical warfare agent (see Chapter 25). It is a common toxic exposure in fires from the combustion of many materials. Iatrogenic intoxication can occur during nitroprusside administration. In addition, acetonitrile-based nail remover, pits of pitted fruits, and consumer exposures from food or drug tampering are uncommon but important potential exposures.

Substances

Household Cyanide Substances	
Fumigation	Silver polishes
Fertilizers	Rodenticides
Insecticides	Imported metal cleaning solutions (e.g., among Hmong refugees)

Insecticides*

Thanite (isobornyl thiocyanoacetate)   Lethane 60
Lethane 384

In insecticides containing aliphatic thiocyanates, HCN is liberated by liver enzymes.

Combustible Household Products*

Plastics   Wool or silk
Polyurethane bedding or furniture   Acrylic baths
Nylon carpets   Melamine resin insulation

Combustion of household products can liberate HCN.

Botanical Sources*

Seeds

Apple (chewed)   Peach   Apricot
Plum   Cherry   Almond

Plants

Improperly prepared cassava   Species of linium and prunus   Sorghum
Lima beans   Bamboo sprouts

Potassium cyanide is found in "Coyote Gitter" shells. Cyanoglycosides found in plants and seeds (e.g., amygdalin) may release HCN after ingestion.

Other Sources

- Laetrile, which contains amygdalin, was a cancer "cure" agent popular in the 1980s.
- Nitrile compounds can release cyanide (CN) through liver metabolism.
- Acetonitrile is found in artificial nail remover.
- Propionitrile
- CN salts
- HCN gas
- Nitroprusside (Remember, CN is a metabolite of nitroprusside.)

Industrial Exposures

Electroplating	Metal heat treating
Gold and silver ore extraction	Recovery of metals from x-ray and
Manufacture of dyes	photographic films
Fumigants	Manufacture of pigments
Chelation	Manufacture of nylon
	Insecticides

Toxicity

- CN exposure causes decreased ATP availability by impaired cellular cytochrome oxidase activity. This leads to decreased tissue oxygen use, cellular hypoxia, and lactate production.
- Impaired oxygen availability causes hypoxic injury.
- It also causes direct neurotoxicity.
- Other effects of CN include:
  - Decreased oxidative metabolism
  - Increased glycolysis
  - Decreased γ-aminobutyric acid (GABA) via inhibition of brain glutamic acid decarboxylase
- Damage can occur to the corpus callosum, corpora striata, hippocampus, and substantia nigra.

Clinical Presentation

- Progressive hypoxia and acidosis
- See Box 15-1.
- Classically, the odor of bitter almonds is associated with CN poisoning.

BOX 15-1 ■ CLINICAL PRESENTATION OF CYANIDE TOXICITY

CNS

Headache, anxiety, agitation, confusion, convulsions, lethargy, coma

Cardiovascular

Bradycardia, hypotension

GI

Abdominal pain, nausea and vomiting due to hemorrhagic gastritis

- However, only 40% of the population can smell it.
- Another classic but unreliable finding is cherry-red skin and retina on fundoscopic exam.

Laboratory Evaluation

- Laboratory clues include a high anion-gap metabolic acidosis that does not improve with supportive therapy.
- CN levels are of no immediate value because it takes several days to obtain the results.

Treatment

- Start with ABCs, IVs, high-flow oxygen, thiamine, dextrose, and naloxone.
- If CN is suspected, the antidote kit (formerly Lilly antidote kit) from Eli Lilly and Co. should be administered and at present is the only FDA-approved treatment.
  - The antidote kit uses amyl nitrite, sodium nitrite, and sodium thiosulfate. The kit has a short shelf life due to its amyl nitrite pearls.
  - Because CN has a higher affinity for methemoglobin than hemoglobin, the antidote is to induce a state of methemoglobinemia through administration of nitrites.
    - The goal is to attain a methemoglobin level of 20%–30%.
    - The CN dissociates from the cytochrome oxidase of hemoglobin and binds to methemoglobin, forming **cyanomethemoglobin**. This is combined with a sulfate group to form thiocyanate, a nontoxic compound that is excreted in the urine.
  - Until an IV is established and parenteral nitrites are prepared, crush amyl nitrite pearls into gauze for patient inhalation or place the crushed pearls over an Ambubag intake valve during assisted or mechanical ventilation. This should be done 30 sec out of each minute.
  - High-flow supplemental oxygen should be applied even if oxygen transport and tension are normal. Oxygen has protective effects and potentiates the effects of the antidotal therapy.
- Administer sodium nitrite ($NaNO_2$) as a 3% solution over 15–20 min.
  - The dose is 10 mL for adults and 0.33 mL/kg for children. It should be diluted in 100–150 mL of solution.

- This will induce a methemoglobin level of about 30%.
- The dose must be corrected downward if the patient is known to be anemic.
- A half-dose may be repeated after 30 minutes if there is no response to the first dose.
- Administer sodium thiosulfate ($Na_2S_2O_3$) as a 25% solution. Adult dose is 50 mL, and the pediatric dose is 1.65 mL/kg.
- Anticipate the possibility of lactic acidosis and hypotension due to nitrite therapy, and correct with fluids and vasopressors.
- Sodium bicarbonate is indicated for acidosis.
- Decontamination consists of activated charcoal and possible orogastric lavage if large quantities are ingested, plus removal of clothing and skin irrigation in cutaneous exposures.
- Dicobalt ethylenediaminetetraacetic acid (EDTA) is currently used in Europe. It chelates CN for renal excretion. It is equally effective as the CN antidote kit; however, it has a wider side-effect profile.
- Hydroxocobalamin/thiosulfate is in clinical trials in the United States and is available in France. It binds the cyanyl group from CN, forming the nontoxic compound cyanocobalamin, which is renally excreted.
  - Usually need 4–7 g to treat CN poisoning

Special Considerations

Fire Toxicology

CN toxicity should be suspected in any fire victim being treated for carbon monoxide poisoning who does not respond to 100% oxygen therapy. Unfortunately, the administration of nitrites to treat CN toxicity can impair oxygen deliver and utilization. If the patient has an elevated carboxyhemoglobin level, nitrites may compound the cellular hypoxia.

Sodium Nitroprusside Infusion

- As CN is released by sodium nitroprusside, it forms thiocyanate, which is excreted in the urine. Thiosulfate is required for this reaction, and the body's stores can be depleted with long-term nitroprusside administration.

- Thiosulfate can be added to the nitroprusside dose with 1 g of thiosulfate added to each 100 mg of sodium nitroprusside.
- The mixture is stable for 7 days provided that it is shielded from light, usually with aluminum foil. After 7 days, thiocyanate toxicity can develop in patients with normal renal function (1–2 days in patients with impaired renal function). The treatment of thiocyanate toxicity is to discontinue the infusion and treat renal insufficiency.

Admission Criteria

Admit symptomatic patients after exposure to CN.

Pearls and Pitfalls

- Cyanide may be found in the pits and seeds of common fruits such as apples, peaches, plums, and cherries.
- Cyanide is a metabolite of nitroprusside.
- The cyanide kit contains amyl nitrite, sodium nitrite, and sodium thiosulfate.
- Cyanide and carbon monoxide poisonings occur together frequently in smoke inhalations, and their toxicity is synergistic.

References and Suggested Readings

1. Cyanide. *Micromedex Healthcare Series,* vol 129, expires Sept 2006. Accessed Feb 2005.
2. Kerns W II, Isom G, Kirk MA: Cyanide and hydrogen sulfide. In Goldfrank LR, Flomenaum NE, Lewin NA, et al, eds: *Goldfrank's toxicologic emergencies,* ed 7, New York, 2002, McGraw-Hill, pp 1498-1504.

2. Carbon Monoxide

Overview

Carbon monoxide (CO) is a byproduct of incomplete combustion of carbonaceous fossil fuels. It is a colorless, odorless toxic gas and is the leading cause of poisoning-related morbidity and mortality in the United States. Winter exposures are most common, and CO poisoning should be suspected when multiple individuals within a single household present with flulike symptoms. In most accidental motor vehicle–related CO deaths, the garage door or windows are open but supply inadequate ventilation.

Substances

Smoke inhalation from fires	Automobile exhaust
Propane-powered equipment, especially indoors or in enclosed spaces	Burning of charcoal, wood, or natural gas
Motorized boats	Heaters
	Paint thinners containing methylene chloride

Toxicity

- CO's primary effect is to create an environment of cellular hypoxia by reducing the systemic arterial oxygen content.
  - It does this by preferentially binding reversibly to hemoglobin, forming carboxyhemoglobin (COHb), which is unable to deliver oxygen to tissues.
    - The affinity of CO for hemoglobin is 200 times greater than that of oxygen.
    - In addition, due to a conformational change in the shape of the hemoglobin molecule, COHb shifts the oxyhemoglobin dissociation curve to the left, impairing oxygen release to tissues.
- There is also preliminary evidence that CO acts independently as an intracellular toxin.
- Free radical formation leads to cellular injury.
- Children and infants have a greater sensitivity to CO poisoning due to a higher metabolic rate.

Clinical Presentation

- The severity of symptoms is dependent on the concentration, duration, comorbidities, and susceptibility of the individual to CO.
  - As expected, the most oxygen-sensitive organs (CNS and cardiovascular) are the most affected by CO poisoning.
  - See Box 15-2.

> **BOX 15-2 ■ SIGNS AND SYMPTOMS OF CARBON MONOXIDE POISONING**
>
> **Nonspecific initial symptoms**
>
> Headache, nausea, dizziness, vomiting
>
> **More severe poisoning**
>
> Syncope, seizures or coma, confusion, pulmonary edema, respiratory failure, bowel incontinence, death
> Cherry-red skin and cutaneous bullae (less frequent or postmortem effects)
>
> **Severe cardiovascular effects**
>
> PVCs, myocardial infarction, dysrhythmias, cardiac arrest, hypotension
> May complain of palpitations
>
> **Other findings**
>
> Myonecrosis, lactic acidosis, retinal hemorrhage

- Nonspecific symptoms are frequently misdiagnosed as viral illnesses.
- Hypotension may accompany severe symptoms due to the vasodilatory effects of CO.
- *Using carboxyhemoglobin levels to determine degree of toxicity is unreliable.* The COHb level only corresponds roughly with symptoms, and in general, stratification of patient's severity based on COHb level requires clinical correlation.

Laboratory Evaluation

- A COHb blood determination is the most useful diagnostic test; however, its measurement should not delay treatment.
  - COHb is misinterpreted for oxyhemoglobin by pulse oximetry, thereby falsely elevating the oxygen saturations by the amount of COHb present.
- In an urban environment, nonsmokers typically have COHb levels of 1%–2% due to automobile exhaust.
- Tobacco smoke contains 4% CO, and smokers typically have a COHb level of 4%–9%.
- Again, the COHb level only corresponds roughly with symptoms, and in general, stratification of patients severity based on COHb level requires clinical correlation.
  - A prolonged exposure to low levels of CO can cause symptoms with low or normal serum levels.

- A lactate determination and ABG are useful in severe poisonings and help determine the severity of poisoning if treatment has started before the patient's arrival at the hospital.
- Neuroimaging is reserved for patients with an unclear diagnosis or those who respond poorly to treatment.
- ECG, troponin, CK

Treatment

- Immediate attention is to the ABCs.
- The antidote for CO poisoning is 100% oxygen delivered immediately, either by endotracheal tube or nonrebreather mask.
- See Table 15-1.
  - On room air oxygen, the half-life of COHb is 320 min.
  - Administration of 100% oxygen reduces the half-life to 80 min.
  - At 3 atmospheres, 100% oxygen reduces the half-life to 23 min.
- Hypotension should be treated with IV fluids and vasopressors as needed.
- Treatment of CO poisoning is associated with a rebound phenomenon. In addition to hemoglobin, myoglobin (particularly cardiac) binds CO. Due to increased affinity, disassociation from myoglobin is slower than hemoglobin. As a result, a rebound effect can be observed, with a delayed elevation of COHb level when disassociated myoglobin CO binds to hemoglobin.

Hyperbaric Oxygen

- Hyperbaric oxygen (HBO) is the inhalation of oxygen at a pressure greater than 1 atmosphere. By creating an environment of high oxygen tension, HBO dissolves oxygen into the hemoglobin molecule to meet the body's increased meta-

Table 15-1 TREATMENT AND ELIMINATION HALF-LIFE OF CARBON MONOXIDE

Treatment	COHb Half-Life
Room air	320 min
100% oxygen	80 min
HBO at 3 atmospheres	23 min

bolic needs. This increases the amount of oxygen available to tissues and therefore accelerates the dissolution of CO from the hemoglobin molecule.

- HBO decreases the half-life of CO poisoning to 23 min at 3 atmospheres and increases the dissolved oxygen content tenfold. In contrast to normobaric oxygen, hyperbaric oxygen prevents lipid peroxidation, which may prevent ischemic reperfusion injury.
- HBO should be used when serious signs and symptoms are present, regardless of COHb levels.
    - This treatment, however, is not without controversy due to conflicting data in the limited clinical trials. It has not been firmly established that HBO therapy improves survival or decreases neuropsychologic sequelae.
- Indications for HBO treatment (Box 15-3)
    - Patients treated with normobaric oxygen therapy for 2 to 4 hr with persistent neurologic symptoms, including headache, ataxia, or confusion, should be referred for HBO therapy.
    - Fetal hemoglobin binds CO more securely than hemoglobin A. This results in a significantly slower rate of disassociation than in the mother and requires five times the length of oxygen therapy.

Special Considerations

Pregnancy

- Fetal COHb levels continue to rise for several hours after maternal levels have peaked and will rise to a level 10% higher than maternal levels.
- Fetal hemoglobin binds CO more securely than hemoglobin A. This results in a significantly slower rate of disassociation than in the mother and requires five times the length of oxygen therapy.
- Pregnancy presents difficulties in CO poisoning due to the effects of the exposure and risks of available treatments.

Box 15-3 Indications for HBO Treatment	
Syncope	Coma
Seizure	Any focal neurologic deficits
COHb levels ≥25%	COHb level ≥15% if pregnant
Acute myocardial infarction (AMI)	Ventricular dysrhythmias
Persistent neurologic symptoms following 100% O_2 treatment	

- After severe maternal poisonings, there is a high incidence of fetal CNS damage and stillbirth.
- Unfortunately, maternal COHb levels are not indicative of fetal hemoglobin or tissue CO levels.
- This relates in part due to slower CO absorption and elimination of the fetal circulation when compared with the adult circulation.
  - Theoretic models predict that CO elimination from the fetus will take five times longer than maternal CO elimination. HBO therapy, however, is not without risk, and there are conflicting data as to the risk of perinatal complications in both minor and significant exposures.
  - The exact COHb level to treat a pregnant patient with HBO is difficult to determine without maternal symptoms or evidence of fetal distress.

Admission Criteria

- Patients with severe toxicity
  - Seizures, coma, resuscitated cardiac arrest
  - Acidemia
  - Acute MI or evidence of myocardial injury
  - Ventricular dysrhythmias
  - Any neurologic deficits

Pearls and Pitfalls

- Fetal hemoglobin binds CO more securely than hemoglobin A. This results in a significantly slower rate of disassociation than in the mother and requires five times the length of oxygen therapy.
- The most common long-term effects are memory impairment and personality deterioration. For this reason, all patients should undergo psychometric testing as outpatients.
- Chronic neuropsychiatric symptoms of CO poisoning are common and are not always directly related to the severity of the exposure.
- In addition to CO poisoning, HBO theoretically has a role in the treatment in cyanide (CN), hydrogen sulfide (H_2S), carbon tetrachloride (CCl_4), and methylene chloride (CH_2Cl_2).
- Methylene chloride is a compound contained in paint thinners whose vapors are absorbed by inhalation. Once in the systemic circulation, it is converted to CO by the liver.

- Pets may be more severely affected due to their smaller size and higher metabolic rates. Illness in both pets and owners can be a clue to CO poisoning.

References and Suggested Readings

1. Tomaszewski C: Carbon monoxide. In Goldfrank LR, Flomenaum NE, Lewin NA, et al, eds: *Goldfrank's toxicologic emergencies,* ed 7, New York, 2002, McGraw-Hill.
2. Tomaszewski C: Carbon monoxide. In Ford MD, Delaney MA, Ling LJ, Erickson T, eds: *Clinical toxicology,* Philadelphia, 2001, WB Saunders.
3. Weaver LK, Hopkins RO, Chan KJ, et al: Hyperbaric oxygen for acute carbon monoxide poisoning, *N Engl J Med* 347:1057-1067, 2002.

3. Chloramine

Overview

Chloramines are chlorinated nitrogen compounds that cause rapid injury by inhalation. Monochloramine (NH_2Cl) is the most common; however, dichloramine ($NHCl_2$) is also toxic. The most common exposure is from mixing ammonia with bleach for cleaning purposes.

Substances

Products containing chlorine bleach mixed with products containing ammonia

Toxicity

When the chloramine gas is inhaled, the mucosal water creates hypochlorous acid–ammonia gas and oxygen-free radicals.

Clinical Presentation

Generally, exposures to low concentrations of chloramines produce only mild respiratory symptoms. However, deaths have been reported from prolonged exposure to the gas formed from mixing sodium hypochlorite bleach and ammonia for bathroom cleaning.

- The majority of patients will have resolution of symptoms within 6 hr; 5%–10% may have symptoms for more than 6 hr after exposure.
  - Shortness of breath
  - Wheezing
  - Cough
  - Chest pain and burning
- Patients with preexisting chronic respiratory problem as well as an upper respiratory tract infection at the time of exposure may have more severe respiratory symptoms and require admission.
- Toxic pneumonitis
- Eye irritation and tearing

Laboratory Evaluation

- ABGs in severely symptomatic patients
- Chest x-ray in patients with symptoms or those with abnormal findings on examination. (This is rarely positive at the time of presentation.)

Treatment

- Oxygen
- Bronchodilators
- Consider steroid therapy in patients with severe respiratory distress and those requiring admission.

Admission Criteria

- Patients requiring treatment for pulmonary complaints (i.e., nebs)
- Most of the patients can safely be discharged after initial ED treatment and evaluation and given appropriate follow-up to be sure they are improving.

Pearls and Pitfalls

- Radiograph findings may lag behind clinical symptoms.
- Ammonia and bleach is one of the common household mixtures.
- Symptoms may occur late.

References and Suggested Readings

1. Hery M, Gerber JM, Hecht G, et al: Exposure to chloramines in a green salad processing plant, *Ann Occup Hyg* 42:437-451, 1998.
2. Mrvos R, Dean BS, Krenzelok EP: Home exposures to chlorine/chloramine gas: review of 216 cases, *South Med J* 86:654-657, 1993.

4. Hydrogen Sulfide

Overview

Hydrogen sulfide (H_2S) is a nonflammable, colorless gas that is heavier than air. It therefore accumulates in low-lying areas and confined spaces. It is an irritating gas that has a "rotten egg" smell; however, olfactory fatigue occurs at high concentrations, eliminating the early warning signs of exposure. Rescuers without proper protective equipment frequently become poisoned.

Substances

H_2S is a natural gas found in crude oil, volcanic gas, sewers, hot springs, and manure pits.

Decomposition of organic matter: manure pits, sewers	Oil wells and petroleum refineries: crude oil and natural gas
Paper mills	Smelters, tanning processes
Natural springs and volcanic gas	Wastewater treatment

Toxicity

- H_2S is a cytochrome oxidase inhibitor, similar to cyanide.
- Forms SulfHgb but not at a level predictive of morbidity

- Decreased tissue oxygen use leads to cellular hypoxia and lactate production.
- Collapse is typically seen with concentrations of 750–1000 ppm, but concentrations as low as 250 ppm can cause chronic symptoms.
- Olfactory fatigue can occur at 100 ppm.
- The U.S. Occupational Safety and Health Administration (OSHA) defines the maximal workplace concentration of H_2S as 20 ppm.

Clinical Presentation

- H_2S causes CNS and pulmonary symptoms.
- Known for its "knockdown effect" whereby unconsciousness can occur after inhaling a single breath (750–1000 ppm).
- Knockdown is likely due to toxic effects on the CNS respiratory center.
- Pulmonary symptoms are also caused by pulmonary edema due to irritation of the terminal bronchial membranes.

Toxicity at Lower Concentrations	
Headache	Nausea
Vomiting	Fatigue

CNS Toxicity	
Dizziness	Lack of coordination
Agitation	Somnolence

- Pulmonary Findings
  - Respiratory depression at H_2S levels of 1000 ppm
  - Pulmonary edema and acute respiratory distress syndrome (ARDS)
  - Pneumonia from impaired ciliary action
- Delayed symptoms are typically neuropsychiatric.
  - Hearing dysfunction
  - Keratoconjunctivitis ("gas eye")
  - Amnesia and CNS depression
  - Motor dysfunction
- A sulfur or rotten-egg odor may be on the patient's clothing,

skin, and breath or even may be noticed emanating from tubes of the patient's blood.
- Thiosulfate formation is the body's main detoxification pathway.
  - Thiosulfate is excreted in the urine.

Laboratory Evaluation

- Sulfhemoglobin levels are not clinically predictive.
- Urinary thiosulfate levels can be used to monitor the extent of exposure of high-risk workers.
- ABGs, electrolytes, CBC
- Chest radiograph

Treatment

- Immediate removal from exposure by rescuer wearing appropriate protective equipment
  - Rescuers have been poisoned by performing mouth-to-mouth on the victim.
- Supportive care and 100% oxygen
  - ABCs
  - Emergency medicine safety net: IV-O_2-Monitor
  - Dextrose if hypoglycemic; thiamine and naloxone depending on clinical presentation
- Induce methemoglobinemia with sodium nitrite.
  - H_2S has a greater affinity for methemoglobin than for cytochrome oxidase.
  - Goal for MetHgb level is 20%–30%. Rapid improvement is expected.
  - Use same dosing as in CN poisoning for adults and children.
  - It is not necessary to use the sodium thiosulfate in the CN kit.
- Sodium bicarb to correct acidosis
- Hyperbaric oxygen therapy has been tried but not proven to be beneficial.

Special Considerations

Contamination of clothing and skin.
  - Remember to wear protective equipment to decontaminate.

Admission Criteria

Admit patients with loss of consciousness, pulmonary findings, and required field resuscitation.

Pearls and Pitfalls

- Coins in the patient's pocket may be darkened from H_2S.
- There is usually more than one victim. The usual scenario is that victim #1 goes into the sewer and does not come out. Victim #2 goes in to rescue victim #1 and does not come out. Usually, the third person wisely calls 911 and avoids the fate of the two coworkers.
- Rescuers performing mouth-to-mouth breathing on a victim may become poisoned.
- H_2S causes a "knockdown effect" at levels of 1000 ppm.
- Olfactory fatigue occurs at 100 ppm, causing the patient to lose the primary warning signal—being able to smell the gas.

References and Suggested Readings

1. Gabbay DS, De Roos F, Perrone J: Twenty-foot fall averts fatality from massive hydrogen sulfide exposure, *J Emerg Med* 20:141-144, 2001.
2. Kerns W II, Isom G, Kirk MA: Cyanide and hydrogen sulfide. In Goldfrank LR, Flomenaum NE, Lewin NA, eds: *Goldfrank's toxicologic emergencies,* ed 7, New York, 2002, McGraw-Hill, pp 1504-1507.
3. Milby TH, Baselt RC: Hydrogen sulfide poisoning: clarification of some controversial issues, *Am J Ind Med* 35:192-195, 1999.

Chapter 16

Snakes and Spiders

Scott Cameron

1. Snakes

Overview

Forty-five thousand snakebites occur annually in the United States; 300,000 to 400,000 bites occur worldwide. In the United States, 7000 to 8000 snakebites are from venomous snakes, causing 5 to 15 deaths annually. About 25% to 50% of bites are "dry bites," meaning there are fang marks but no venom or envenomation. Of the 120 species of snakes in the United States, only 26 are venomous. Two families of venomous snakes are native to the United States: Elapidae (coral snakes) and Crotalinae (pit vipers [e.g., rattlesnakes, water moccasins, copperheads]). Pit vipers account for 95% of all envenomations. In addition to native species, patients occasionally present with envenomation from exotic snakes kept as pets. The clinician should contact the local poison control center, herpetologists, or local zoos for antivenom. The *Antivenom Index,* published by the American Zoo and Aquarium Association and the American Association of Poison Control Centers, lists the locations, amounts, and various types of antivenom.

Species

Pit Vipers (Crotalinae*)

- Rattlesnakes, cottonmouths, water moccasins
- Mojave rattlesnake: only pit viper with neurotoxic venom. May cause severe and delayed neurologic symptoms such as severe weakness or respiratory paralysis.
- Characteristic, heat-sensitive "pit" located midway between the eye and nostril
- Elliptical pupil, triangular head

Formerly Crotalidae.

Coral Snakes (Elapidae)

- Eastern coral snake: AR, NC, SC, FL, LA, GA, MS, TX
- Western coral snake: AZ, NM. No deaths reported
- Often confused with the king snake species
- Usually shy, reclusive; will only bite if provoked
- "Red on yellow, kill a fellow, red on black, venom lack"
- Unlike pit viper bites, local damage is usually mild and does not correlate with severity of envenomation.
- All confirmed coral snake envenomations are defined as severe and require antivenom.

Toxicity

Pit Vipers

- Venom consists of proteolytic enzymes and anticoagulant esterases. Basically, it attempts to digest the victim.
- Mojave neurotoxin blocks the N-type calcium channels.
  - Mojave A neurotoxin
  - Mojave B hemotoxin and cytotoxin (found in the area of Phoenix, AZ)

Coral Snakes

- Elapidae venom is a potent neurotoxin and may cause paresthesias, weakness, cranial nerve dysfunction, confusion, fasciculations, and lethargy.

- α-neurotoxin binds to postsynaptic acetylcholine receptor and causes a nondepolarizing neuromuscular blockade (i.e., curare).
- β-neurotoxin increases the release of ACh and then inhibits the release of ACh (i.e., botulinum toxin).

Clinical Presentation

Pit Vipers

- Edema: Usually presents within 1 hr in moderate-severe bites. Can be pronounced. Spreads centrally over 8–24 hr. Mark the leading edge of edema with a pen every 30 min.
  - Compartment syndrome can develop, although this is rare and probably overdiagnosed. It is often difficult to separate the local effects of the envenomation from compartment syndrome because both may cause pallor, paresthesias, swelling, and severe pain.
  - Monitor capillary refill and consider consulting a surgeon if elevated compartment pressures refractory to antivenom are strongly suspected.
- Ecchymosis, petechiae, and hemorrhagic bullae often develop.
- Pain is often immediate and severe.
- Systemic effects: May cause nausea, vomiting, paresthesias, dizziness, and diaphoresis. Severe envenomations may cause hypotension, rhabdomyolysis and renal failure, mental status changes, and respiratory distress.
- Coagulopathy: Increase in PT, PTT, thrombocytopenia, and hemolysis may occur. Disseminated intravascular coagulation (DIC) may occur in severe cases.
- Head and trunk envenomations are generally more serious than extremity bites.
- Children: Because of their smaller size and weight, they are at a higher risk of severe envenomation.
- Envenomations are graded as minimal, moderate, and severe (Box 16-1).

Coral Snakes

- Often mild local findings
- Elapidae venom is a potent neurotoxin and may cause paresthesias, weakness, cranial nerve dysfunction, confusion, fasciculations, and lethargy.
  - Diplopia, ptosis, and dysarthria are common early symptoms.

BOX 16-1 ▪ GRADING THE SEVERITY OF SNAKEBITE ENVENOMATION

Minimal

Moderate pain, swelling, and erythema confined to bite area. No systemic signs or symptoms. No coagulation abnormalities.

Moderate

More severe pain; extension of edema and erythema toward trunk; involves less than entire extremity. Systemic signs and symptoms may include tachycardia, mild hypotension, or perioral paresthesias. Laboratory findings may show coagulation abnormalities, but no evidence of bleeding is noted. Bad.

Severe

Severe pain, erythema, and edema that involves entire extremity and may reach and involve trunk. Airway compromise is possible. Early systemic involvement with nausea, vomiting, muscle cramping and pain, and tachycardia. Significant laboratory abnormalities include rhabdomyolysis, severe coagulation abnormalities; renal failure may be seen. Seizures, shock, hemorrhage, coma, and death may occur. Really bad.

- Patients die because of respiratory paralysis. **Early and aggressive airway management is vital.**
- Symptoms may be delayed by 8 to 12 hr.
- Nausea, vomiting, and salivation are also common.

Laboratory Evaluation

- CBC, coagulation studies, DIC panel
- CK, renal function, UA
- Type and crossmatch in severe envenomations

Treatment

Prehospital Management

- Remove the individual from the vicinity of snake.
- Immobilize the bite site just below heart level.
- Minimize all physical activity (this diminishes absorption of venom).
  - Consider venom extractor if it can be applied immediately.
  - **Do not incise bite marks.**
- Transport immediately to nearest hospital.

ED Management

- ABCs, IV hydration
- Antivenom indicated for moderate to severe envenomations
  - Two kinds of antivenom: Wyeth polyvalent antivenom and CroFab
  - Wyeth: made with horse serum; higher rate of anaphylaxis and serum sickness
    - Skin test recommended in moderate envenomations (if truly severe, infuse without skin test; it is worth the risk)
    - Intracutaneous injection of 0.02–0.03 mL of a 1:10 dilution of horse serum or antivenom is recommended in the package insert. A positive test result is the development of a wheal within 5–30 min.
    - Skin testing is unreliable. Always start the infusion **Very slowly,** even with a negative skin test.
    - If positive skin test and envenomation progresses, pretreat with Benadryl, steroids, and possibly even SQ epinephrine and attempt to infuse the antivenom slowly.
  - Reconstitute the antivenom in 10 mL of NS (it may take 20–60 min of continuous mixing). Then redilute 1:2 with NS.
- Start infusion very slowly: 0.5 mL/min for first 10 min.
  - Moderate envenomation: 5–10 vials
  - Severe envenomation: 10–20 vials
  - CroFab: Crotalinae polyvalent immune Fab (ovine)
  - Highly purified, sheep-derived antivenom; contains venom-specific Fab fragments that bind and neutralize venom
  - Reportedly has a much lower rate of acute reactions and serum sickness. However, a recent study showed 19% acute reactions (versus 20%–25% with Wyeth) and 23% serum sickness (versus 50%–75% with Wyeth antivenom).
  - Some evidence of recurrent coagulopathy in patients treated with CroFab; may present up to 1 week following treatment
  - FDA-approved for treatment of minimal to moderate envenomations
  - Skin testing not required
  - Initial dose: 4–6 vials. Repeat in 1 hr if further progression of symptoms. Some recommend 2 units every 6 hr for 3 doses after initial dose.
  - As with Wyeth antivenom, start infusion slowly and monitor closely for anaphylaxis.

- Confining the spread of venom to an extremity with tourniquets actually increases morbidity because of greater tissue damage. Cryotherapy and electrocautery are bad ideas.

Coral Snakes (Elapidae)

Prehospital Management
- As above
  - Transport immediately to nearest hospital.

ED Management
- Monitor vital signs and neurologic symptoms carefully and frequently.
- Intubate if any evidence of respiratory compromise or bulbar muscle involvement.
- Antivenom indicated for all confirmed Eastern coral snake bites (Western: no antivenom).
  - 3–5 vials diluted in 500 mL of NS over 30–60 min after negative skin test.
  - Monitor for and treat anaphylaxis aggressively.

Special Considerations

- Pediatrics
  - Due to their smaller size, children are more susceptible to severe envenomation.
- Pregnancy
- Start antivenom in pregnant women when indicated, but monitor the fetus during treatment.
- Novice herpetologists and professional snake handlers
  - These brave souls may have repeated bites and eventually develop an allergy to the antivenom after multiple treatments.

Admission Criteria

- Admit all patients with confirmed coral snake bites for careful observation.
- If no evidence of envenomation, observe for 6 hr.
- If evidence of local pain or erythema, observe for 12 hr.
- Admit all patients with progressive symptoms to an ICU.

- Also admit any patient who has been bitten by a Mojave rattlesnake or an exotic snake.

Pearls and Pitfalls

- Do not handle snakes, even if they are dead. Significant envenomations have occurred from handling the decapitated heads of seemingly dead snakes.
- Elapidae = coral snakes = neurotoxin.
- "Red on yellow, kill a fellow; red on black, venom lack."
  - The victim commonly has difficulty remembering this mnemonic or heeding its intended warning when intoxicated and attempts to interact or "play" with the snake.
- Consider early intubation and antivenom if significant Elapidae envenomation.
- Crotalidae (Crotalinae) = pit vipers = local damage.
- All severe envenomations were at one time minimal envenomations that progressed. Observe all bites carefully.

References and Suggested Readings

1. Gold BS, Dart RC, Barish RA, et al: Bites of venomous snakes, *N Engl J Med* 2002;347:347-356.
2. McKinney PE. Out-of-hospital and interhospital management of crotaline snakebite. *Ann Emerg Med* 2002;37:168-174.
3. Roberts JR, Otten EJ: Snakes and other reptiles. In Goldfrank LR, Flomenaum NE, Lewin NA, et al, eds: *Goldfrank's toxicologic emergencies,* ed 7, New York, 2002, McGraw-Hill,
4. Sullivan JB, Wingert WA, Norris RL. North American venomous reptile bites. In Auerbach PS, ed: *Wilderness medicine: management of wilderness and environmental emergencies,* ed 7. St. Louis, 1995, Mosby-Year Book, pp 680-709.

2. Spiders

Overview

There are 30,000 different species of spiders worldwide. Nearly all have venom, but most species are not harmful to people because their fangs cannot penetrate human skin. Only 50 species have been implicated in significant envenomations in the United States. Most of these cases involved mild local symptoms and pruritis.

▣ Species

▣ *Loxosceles*

- Brown; 8–15 mm long; long legs
- Characteristic dark violin–shaped mark on cephalothorax
- Nocturnal; prefer warm, dry indoor areas such as sheds, cellars, and abandoned buildings
- 5 species associated with necrotic loxoscelism: *L. reclusa* (**brown recluse—#1**), *L. refuscens, L. arizona, L. unicolor, L. laeta*

▣ *Latrodectus* (**Black Widow**)

- Common worldwide
- 5 species in United States, particularly in the western and southern states
- *L. mactans mactans* = black widow
- Black, shiny, 2–2.5 cm with long legs
- Female is venomous; male is small and harmless
- Found in basements, woodpiles, and garages

▣ Toxicity

Loxosceles

- Causes severe cutaneous necrosis; infrequently may cause systemic reactions with coagulopathy, renal failure, hemolysis, death
- 5 species associated with necrotic loxoscelism: *L. reclusa* (**brown recluse— #1**), *L. refuscens, L. arizona, L. unicolor, L. laeta*
- Venom is hemolytic and cytotoxic. Serves to enzymatically digest its prey. Contains sphingomyelinase D, a potent cytotoxin.
  - Causes tissue necrosis by leukocyte aggregation and platelet plugging of arterioles and venules.

Latrodectus

- Potent neurotoxic venom causes severe muscle spasms.
- Venom (α-lactotoxin) is neurotoxic and causes acetylcholine and neuroepi release at synaptic junction.

▣ Clinical Presentation

Loxosceles

- Local symptoms are immediately affected: stinging sensation, then pruritis.
- Bite site becomes red, edematous, and then acentral violaceous area appears (necrosis), often with rings separated by white areas of vasospasm ("red, white, and blue" or "bull's-eye" lesion).
- In severe cases, hemorrhagic bullae or vesicles arise within 1–3 days.
- Eschar forms and then sloughs away in several weeks, leaving an ulcer that may persist for months.
- Systemic involvement is less common and does not correlate with severity of ulcer. It occurs most often in children.
- Nausea/vomiting/hemolysis, fever, thrombocytopenia, renal failure
- 8 deaths have been reported.

Lactrodectus

- Initial bite may be painful or may not be noticed.
- Local reaction is often trivial, such as a small papule or punctum.
- Some cases progress to dramatic neuromuscular symptoms over the next 30–60 min, but generally within 6 hr.
- Spasm, muscle cramps, and rigidity of major muscle groups begin at the site of bite and then spread.
  - Patient may develop "facies lactrodectus."
- Severe pain, fasciculations, weakness, vomiting, diaphoresis, priapism, rare rhabdomyolysis
- Involvement of abdominal muscles may mimic peritonitis.
- Hypertension with or without seizures in older adults or previously hypertensive patients (often severe)
- Children: intractable crying
- Pregnant women: Bite could induce contractions and premature labor.
- Symptoms subside over several hours but may recur for days to 1 week.

▣ Laboratory Evaluation

CBC and coagulation studies in cases of severe systemic reactions.

Treatment

Loxosceles

Treatment depends on severity. All wounds require tetanus prophylaxis, appropriate analgesia, and daily wound care.
* RICE, ice packs 15 min/hr
* Controversial treatments for severe local necrosis
    * Wound excision: No; worse outcome
    * HBO: Little to no evidence of benefit
    * Dapsone: No controlled human studies; inhibits chemotactic migration of neutrophils; controversial; may cause hemolysis if G6PD deficient; so check before starting. Only consider for severe local necrosis.
    * Steroids: No proven benefit
    * Topical nitroglycerin: Does not work
    * Antivenom: Only available for *L. laeta* (South America)
    * Beer: Personal favorite; cannot hurt
* No antibiotics unless infected
* Patients with significant local symptoms or any systemic complaints: Draw CBC, coagulation profile, urinalysis, renal function tests.

Lactrodectus

* Supportive: ABCs
* Local wound care and tetanus
* Treatment of spasms with narcotics and benzodiazepines
* Calcium gluconate: Shown to be ineffective. Stick with benzodiazepines.
* Severe HTN: Control with labetalol, nitroprusside
* Antivenom: Horse serum (risk of anaphylaxis is 0.5%)—use in severe envenomations with respiratory arrest, pregnancy, seizures, uncontrolled HTN.

Special Considerations

* Pediatric and older adult patients
    * More likely to have coagulopathy and hemolysis

Admission Criteria

- Admit all patients with systemic symptoms.
- Consider plastic surgery referral for all severe local reactions.

Lactrodectus

Admit all symptomatic children, pregnant women, and hypertensive adults.

Pearls and Pitfalls

- Recluse = necrose.
- Necrotic arachnidism can be caused by many American spiders. It can be confused with third-degree burns, herpes simplex, decubitus ulcers, and pyoderma gangrenosum.
- *Lactrodectus*
  - Minimal local reaction (in contrast to recluse). If it is swollen, it is probably not a black widow bite.
  - Severe muscle spasms and pain within 1 hr. Memory aid: "Latro-wrecked-us" or "Latro-pect-us" (as in "pectoralis") or even "Latro-WreckedOurPect-us."
- **Benzodiazepines**

References and Suggested Readings

1. Rash LD, Kodgson WC: Pharmacology and biochemistry of spider venoms, *Toxicon* 2002;40:225-254.
2. Hampton R Sr: Spider bites. http://www.emedicine.com/oph/topic652.htm. Accessed Feb 15, 2002.

Chapter 17

Toxic Foods

STEVE WANDERSEE

1. Ciguatera Fish Poisoning

Overview

Ciguatera (the Spanish word for "poisonous snail") is the most common of the nonbacterial fish-borne poisonings. Ciguatera toxin is found in reef fish that consume certain types of dinoflagellates or algae. Consumption of these reef fish found in warm water reefs causes ciguatera poisoning in humans. Worldwide transportation of fish in recent years has caused ciguatera poisoning to be found anywhere in the world.

Gambierdiscus toxicus is the primary dinoflagellate that produces ciguatera toxin. Other toxins produced are maitotoxin and scaritoxin.

Sources

Amberjack	Barracuda	Cinnamon
Coral trout	Dolphin fish	Eel
Emperor	Grouper	Kingfish
Paddletail	Parrot fish	Red snapper
Reef cord	Sea bass	Spanish mackerel
Squirrel fish	Sturgeon fish	Yankee whiting

Toxicity

- Ciguatoxin and other similar toxins are **heat stable** and therefore are unaffected by cooking, temperature, and gastric acid.
- They are also lipid soluble, thus the presence of the toxin does not affect odor, color, or taste of the fish.
- The larger the affected fish, the more toxins present.

Clinical Presentation

- Onset of symptoms is usually in 1 hr but may occur up to 3 days after ingestion.
- Neurologic symptoms have persisted for **months** in rare cases.
- Common symptoms
  - Increased salivation, chills, pruritis, dyspnea, and neck stiffness
  - Nausea, vomiting, diarrhea, and abdominal pain are usually present.
  - Myalgia and arthralgias are also common.
  - Dysuria, urethritis, painful ejaculation, and dyspareunia in the *unaffected* partner have been reported.
- Neurologic symptoms seem to be the most bothersome and persist for a longer period of time.
  - Headache, weakness, vertigo, and ataxia are usually present.
  - Cranial nerve palsy, visual hallucinations, seizures, and coma have been noted in more serious cases.
- Paradoxical temperature reversal (i.e., cold objects feel hot, and hot objects feel cold) can occur.
- Patients have also reported lingual and perioral paresthesias as well as paresthesias of the extremities.
- Dental pain or patient reports of extremely loose tooth sensations have been noted.
- Cardiovascular symptoms include bradycardia, hypotension, and arrhythmias.
- Respiratory depression, bronchospasm, and even respiratory failure can occur.

Differential Diagnoses

- Scombroid and tetrodotoxin (see the next sections)
- Mushroom, amatoxin or disulfiram-like toxins, Gyromitra toxin

- Drug toxicity: beta-blockers, calcium channel blockers, carbamazepine, disulfiram, isoniazid, lithium, and phenytoin
- Mercury and arsenic toxicity
- Snake envenomations: cobra, sea snake, and coral

Laboratory Evaluation

- ECG may show cardiac involvement.
- Electrolytes should be done if vomiting and diarrhea are present.
- An ELISA test is available to detect ciguatera toxin but may not be stocked by all labs.

Treatment

- Treatment is usually supportive and pertains to the organ system affected. Monitoring should include vital signs.
- Dehydration should be treated with IV fluid replacement.
- Antiemetics will control nausea and vomiting.
- Antihistamines can be used for pruritis.
- Activated charcoal has proven helpful if given within 3 hr of ingestion.
- Mannitol or other osmotic diuretics can be used to treat neurologic symptoms and have been found to be most effective if given early in the course of the illness.
- Serotonin and norepinephrine reuptake inhibitors may also help with neurologic symptoms as well as with pruritis.

Special Considerations

Consumption of any fish product or shellfish may exacerbate symptoms. Other **foods to avoid are nuts and oils** as well as **alcohol**. Subsequent exposure usually is associated with more persistent neurologic symptoms.

Admission Criteria

Admit patients with severe symptoms such as hallucinations, seizures, or coma.

Pearls and Pitfalls

- Reversal of hot and cold sensation is pathognomonic for ciguatera poisoning.
- Ciguatoxin is heat stable.
- The larger the fish, the more toxic.

References and Suggested Readings

1. Editorial staff: Ciguatera Fish Poisoning. Poisindex® Syst em. Thomson Micromedex, Greenwood Village, Co. Vol. 128. Expired June 2006.
2. Thompson A: Toxicity, Ciguatera. http://www.emedicine.com/emerg/topic100.htm. Last updated: Jan 3, 2006. Accessed June 27, 2006.

2. Tetrodotoxin Poisoning

Overview

Poisoning occurs after ingestion of several different species of puffer fish. Poisoning primarily occurs in Japan because the Japanese have a fondness for the puffer fish (a delicacy known as *fugu*). Improper handling of the fish causes the problem. The toxin is present in the skin, viscera, and gonads of the fish. Mortality rates have been reported in up to 50% of cases.

Sources

Puffer fish, balloon fish, blowfish, swell fish, toad fish, glove fish
Some salamanders or newts
Blue-ringed octopus
Frogs, gastropods, crabs, and starfish

Toxicity

- Tetrodotoxin acts directly on the sodium ion channel responsible for nerve and muscle excitability.
  - Acts directly on the central and peripheral nervous systems.
- Onset of symptoms is usually within 15 min to several hours.
- The LD50 dose is 8μg/kg. Death can occur within 4–6 hr.

◼ Clinical Presentation

- Common symptoms include lip, tongue, and facial and extremity paresthesias.
- Both hypotension and hypertension have been noted.
- Paralysis can occur and is often rapid in onset.
- Death is usually secondary to respiratory muscle paralysis.
- Peripheral paralysis, blurred vision, difficulty speaking, increased salivation, nausea, and vomiting are usually present.
- Seizures and coma have been reported.
- Cardiac arrhythmias and bradycardia have been noted.

Differential Diagnoses

- Scombroid, ciguatera and shellfish poisoning
- Guillain-Barré syndrome
- Octopus envenomation
- Botulism
- Gastroenteritis

◼ Laboratory Evaluation

- Routine monitoring, oxygen, ECG, and electrolytes are indicated.
- Chest radiograph
- CT of the head may be useful in the differential diagnosis.

◼ Treatment

There is no antidote, and so treatment is primarily supportive. Protection of the airway is of primary importance; thus the patient may need endotracheal intubation. Treat abnormal vital signs aggressively.

- Early administration of activated charcoal **may** help.
- Neostigmine 0.5 mg IM in adults and 0.02 mg/kg IV or 0.04 mg/kg IM in pediatric cases have been given with mixed results.

▌ Special Considerations

- Tetrodotoxin has been considered as a potential biological warfare agent that could be placed in drinking water.
- It can be inactivated by 0.5 ppm of chlorine.

▌ Admission Criteria

- Patient with respiratory difficulty, seizure, or dysrhythmias
- ICU admission is indicated. Prognosis is good if patient survives the first 24 hr.
- Symptoms can last up to several days and should be monitored closely.

Pearls and Pitfalls

- Symptoms can begin as soon as 15 min after eating the bad fish.
- Death is usually from respiratory paralysis.
- Puffer fish is served as a delicacy known as *fugu* in Japan; a single serving costs hundreds of dollars. Only trained and licensed chefs may prepare puffer fish in Japan, taking particular care with the gonads, skin, liver, and intestines. Chefs are required to pass a strict written exam and demonstrate their technique by preparing *fugu* and then eating it.

▌ References and Suggested Readings

1. Editorial staff: Tetrodotoxin. Poisindex® System. Thomson Micromedex, Greenwood Village, Co. Vol. 128. Expired June 2006.
2. Benzer TI: Toxicity, Tetrodotoxin. http://www.emedicine.com/emerg/topic576.htm. Last updated Feb 17, 2005. Accessed June 27, 2006.

3. Scombroid Fish Poisoning

▌ Overview

Scombrotoxin *(not "Scrombotoxin")* is the toxin involved in scombroid fish poisoning. This is the second most common toxin in fish, after ciguatera toxin. Consumption of contaminated reef fish causes a histaminelike reaction in humans.

Sources

Dark-meat fish

Tuna, mackerel, skipjack, bonito, marlin

Nonscombroid species

Mahi-mahi, sardine, yellowtail, herring, bluefish

Toxicity

- Scombrotoxin, like ciguatoxin, is *heat stable,* meaning cooking does not deactivate the toxin.
  - The histidine in dark-meat fish is decarboxylated to histamine by bacteria on or in the fish.
- Improperly frozen or excessive thawing of fish has been implicated in this poisoning.

Clinical Presentation

- Onset of symptoms is usually **within 10–60 min** of eating contaminated fish.
- There is a frequent mention of a **sharp peppery or bitter taste** to the fish, but it is not always present.
- Symptoms usually last 3–36 hr.
- Patients present usually with a histaminelike reaction.
  - Flushing or erythema of the skin and angioedema of the face may occur.
  - Palpitations, tachycardia, or asthmalike symptoms are often present.
  - Neurologic symptoms can include headache, anxiety, dizziness, and weakness.
  - Patients often present with nausea, vomiting, and diarrhea.

Differential Diagnoses

- Ciguatera toxin
- Tetrodotoxin
- Anaphylaxis
- Toxic shock syndrome
- Bee and Hymenoptera stings

- Cluster headache
- Allergic reaction
- Niacin reactions

Laboratory Evaluation

- Usually not indicated
- Histamine level can be measured in the suspected fish.
  - Illness is usually associated with a level of 100 mg/100 g of fish.
  - Normal fish levels of histamine are less than 1 mg/100 g of fish.
  - Levels as low as 20 mg/100 g can cause symptoms in some people.

Treatment

- Supportive treatment as indicated may include oxygen, monitoring, and IV access.
- Some recommend administration of activated charcoal if the patient presents early after ingestion and if a large portion of contaminated fish has been ingested.
- Antihistamines are the mainstays of controlling symptoms.
  - Both H1 and H2 blockers have been successful.
  - Treatment with histamine blockade should be for 3–5 days.
- SubQ epinephrine has been administered to patients with asthma-like symptoms.
- Patients must avoid eating fish that has been improperly frozen or thawed.

Special Considerations

- Pediatric and the elderly are especially susceptible to severe symptoms, especially respiratory.

Admission Criteria

Admission is usually not necessary unless severe respiratory symptoms fail to respond to ED treatment.

Pearls and Pitfalls

- Scombroid toxicity is due to ingestion of histamine, not intrinsic histamine from the patient.
- Patient most likely will respond to antihistamines.
- Patients may complain of a sharp peppery taste of the fish.

References and Suggested Readings

1. Editorial staff: Scombroid Fish Poisoning. Poisindex® System. Thomson Micromedex, Greenwood Village, Co. Vol. 128. Expired June 2006.
2. Patrick JD: Toxicity, Scombroid. http://www.emedicine.com/EMERG/topic523.htm. Last updated Nov 15, 2005. Accessed on June 27, 2006.

4. Shellfish Toxicity

Overview

Shellfish toxicity involves the eating of filter-feeding mollusks such as clams, mussels, oysters, and scallops, which accumulate toxins from **dinoflagellates**.

Sources

- All shellfish are potentially toxic.
- Outbreaks are associated with algae blooms called *red tide*, which usually occur in warmer months.

Toxicity

Four primary toxins are involved.

- Saxitoxin associated with paralytic shellfish poisoning (PSP)
- Brevotoxin associated with neurologic shellfish poisoning (NSP)
- Okadaic acid associated with diarrheal shellfish poisoning (DSP)
- Domoic acid associated with amnestic shellfish poisoning (ASP)

Clinical Presentation

Onset of symptoms can be from minutes to hours. Symptoms may persist for weeks.

Paralytic Shellfish Poisoning

- Paresthesias of the lips, tongue, and gingiva are common.
- Patients may also experience the sensation of floating, headache, ataxia, muscle weakness, paralysis, and cranial nerve dysfunction.
- Nausea, vomiting, and diarrhea can occur.
- Death is usually secondary to respiratory paralysis.
- Symptoms present from 3 days to weeks.

Neurologic Shellfish Poisoning

- This is very similar to ciguatera poisoning with its reversal of hot and cold sensations.
- Paresthesias of face and extremities are common.
- Nausea, vomiting, and diarrhea may be present.
- Headache, dizziness, ataxia, vertigo, tremors, and bradycardia have been noted.
- Allergic response is characterized by rhinorrhea, conjunctivitis, bronchospasm, and cough in sensitive individuals who live near shorelines because brevotoxins are aerosolized by the surf.

Diarrheal Shellfish Poisoning

- Primarily nausea, vomiting, and diarrhea, which can last 1–2 days
- Most common in Japan and Europe

Amnestic Shellfish Poisoning

- This is rare.
- Nausea, vomiting, diarrhea, and short-term memory loss have been noted.
- Seizures, coma, hemiparesis, and ophthalmoplegia have been seen in severe toxicity.
- Mortality rate is approximately 3%.

Differential Diagnoses

- Botulism, ciguatera, scombroid toxicity
- Tetrodotoxin
- Organophosphates and phenytoin toxicity

Laboratory Evaluation

There are no useful laboratory tests.

Treatment

- Monitoring, oxygen, and IV access are indicated.
- Fluid replacement because most patients have depleted fluid volumes. Maintain airway. Monitor more severe cases for 24 hr.
- Activated charcoal can be used within 4 hr of ingestion.
- Neostigmine has been used to improve muscle weakness.
- Patients should avoid shellfish from areas that contain red tide. Patients need to be closely observed as long as symptoms persist.

Special Considerations

- Pediatric patients are especially susceptible to saxitoxin.
- Elderly patients tend to have the highest mortality.

Pearls and Pitfalls

- PSP is generally associated with mussels, clams, cockles, and scallops.
- NSP is generally associated with shellfish harvested along the Florida coast and the Gulf of Mexico.
- DSP is generally associated with mussels, oysters, and scallops.
- ASP is generally associated with mussels.

References and Suggested Readings

1. Arnold T: Toxicity, Shellfish. http://www.emedicine.com/emerg/topic528.htm. Last updated March 21, 2006. Accessed on June 27, 2006.
2. Various Shellfish-Associated Toxins. In the Bad bug book: Foodborne pathogenic microorganisms and natural toxins handbook. U.S. Food and Drug Administration, Center for Food Safety & Applied Nutrition. http://www.cfsan.fda.gav/~mow/chap37.html. Last updated june 14, 2006. Accessed on June 27, 2006.
3. Editorial Staff: Shellfish Poisoning. Poisindex® System. Thomson Micromedex, Greenwood Village, CO. Vol. 128.

Special
Tox
Conditions

Conditions caused by overdoses and toxins that will help you effectively and efficiently manage these problems in the ED or on the ward.

Chapter 18

Methemoglobinemia

STEPHANIE WITT

Overview

Methemoglobin is formed from the oxidation of ferrous iron (Fe^{2+}) to ferric iron (Fe^{3+}) within the hemoglobin molecule.

Substances

Common Agents That Produce Methemoglobinemia		
Aniline (dyes, ink)	Lidocaine	Nitroprussid
Benzocaine (teething gels)	Metoclopramide	Nitroglycerin
Chlorates*	Methylene blue	Paraquat
Chloroquine or primaquine	Naphthalene (mothballs)	Phenazopyridine
Dapsone	Nitrates (well water)	Phenol
Dinitrophenol (pesticide)	Nitric oxide	Phenytoin
	Nitrites	Sulfonamides

*Chlorates found in explosives, matches, dyes, weed killers, mouthwash, and weak antiseptics.

Common Causes of Methemoglobinemia by Age Group		
6 months	Older Children	Adolescents and Adults
Most commonly due to severe metabolic acidosis secondary to diarrhea or dehydration Well water nitrates (e.g., well water used to dilute formula) Presentation similar to cyanotic congenital heart disease, but patient has normal cardiopulmonary exam and chest radiographs	Ingestion of dapsone, pyridium, nitroalkene (nail polish remover) Cyanosis occurs shortly after ingestion	Inhalant abuse (volatile nitrates)

▪ Toxicity

- Methemoglobin impairs the ability of hemoglobin to transport O_2 and CO_2, leading to tissue hypoxemia, impaired aerobic respiration, metabolic acidosis, and even death.
- Left shift of the oxygen-hemoglobin dissociation curve, with the result that oxygen is bound more tightly and is poorly released to tissues
- Net positive charge of hemoglobin so that it has a high affinity for negative ions such as cyanide, fluoride, or chloride
- Sometimes accompanied by hemolysis secondary to associated damage to cell

▪ Clinical Presentation

- Tachypnea, tachycardia, cyanosis
- Acute shortness of breath, tachycardia, and cyanosis resemble pulmonary embolism, but evaluation fails to confirm hypoxia, raising the suspicion of methemoglobinemia.
- Symptoms are related to impaired oxygen delivery.
- Severity of symptoms depends on MetHgb level (Table 18-1).
  - Patients with underlying cardiac, pulmonary, or hematologic disease may experience more severe symptoms for a given MetHgb concentration.

Table 18-1 METHEMOGLOBIN LEVELS AND ASSOCIATED SYMPTOMS

Methemoglobin Concentration	% Total Hemoglobin*	Symptoms
<1.5 g/dL	<10	None
1.5–3.0 g/dL	10–20	Cyanosis
3.0–4.5 g/dL	20–30	Anxiety, lightheadedness, headache, tachycardia
4.5–7.5 g/dL	30–50	Fatigue, confusion, dizziness, tachypnea, increased tachycardia
7.5–10.5 g/dL	50–70	Coma, seizures, arrhythmias, acidosis
>10.5 g/dL	>0	Death

Assumes Hgb = 15 g/dL. Patients with lower hemoglobin concentrations may experience more severe symptoms for a given percentage of MetHgb level.

Laboratory Evaluation

- Cyanosis unresponsive to oxygen therapy (with normal cardiopulmonary exam)
- Chocolate-brown blood that does not change color upon exposure to air
- Co-oximetry
  - Direct laboratory measurement of MetHgb
  - Most accurate measurement of actual blood oxygen content
- ABG
  - Arterial blood is a chocolate-brown color.
  - Normal to increased PO_2 levels
  - Normal calculated O_2 saturation (because PO_2 is based on O_2 dissolved in blood not bound to hemoglobin)
- Pulse oximetry
  - Overestimates level of oxygen saturation
  - Usually normal because methemoglobin has absorptive characteristics similar to oxyhemoglobin
  - Significant MetHb levels (>30%) results in $SatO_2$ approaching 85% (maximal $SatO_2$ depression seen if condition is due to methemoglobinemia alone).
  - Saturation gap (difference between measured $SatO_2$ and calculated $SatO_2$) indicates presence of another substance such as MetHgb.

Treatment

- ABCs
- Adequate decontamination with charcoal

- If MetHgb ≥30%, MetHgb ≥20%, and patient is symptomatic or MetHgb ≥10% with other comorbidities:
  - Methylene blue 1–2 mg/kg IV over 3–5 min
  - Repeat 1 mg/kg if cyanosis does not resolve within 1 hr.
  - Dextrose should be administered with methylene blue.
- Other treatments (not standard): cytochrome p-450 inhibitor (cimetidine or ketoconazole), *N*-acetylcysteine, ascorbic acid, hyperbaric oxygen, exchange transfusion

▌ Special Considerations

- **Relapsing methemoglobinemia** (levels decrease with methylene blue but then rebound again to toxic levels) or treatment failure
  - Due to inadequate decontamination and/or ingestion of an agent that produces methemoglobin cyclically (aniline, benzocaine, dapsone)
  - Repeat charcoal.
  - Repeat administration of methylene blue in 1 hr if signs persist, then every 4 hr to maximum dose of 7 mg/kg. (Methylene blue displays toxicity manifested by dyspnea, chest pain, and hemolysis.)
  - Consider congenital enzyme deficiency (MetHgb reductase, G6PD), Hgb M, sulfhemoglobinemia as other possible causes of treatment failure.
- Sulfhemoglobinemia
  - Most drugs that produce methemoglobinemia can also produce sulfhemoglobin in a process where the heme moiety is first oxidized to MetHgb and then covalently bound to sulfur.
  - Symptoms are milder because of decreased affinity for O_2 in remaining unaffected hemoglobin, making O_2 more available to tissues.
  - Symptoms may last 1–6 months, depending on the SulfHgb level.
  - Diagnosed by spectrophotometry or gas chromatography/mass spectrometry.
  - Potassium cyanide test differentiates between MetHgb and SulfHgb: MetHgb will turn bright red when exposed to cyanide. SulfHgb remains dark brown.
  - SulfHgb cannot be reduced: It does not respond to methylene blue or other antidotes.
  - Treatment is supportive. For severe sulfhemoglobinemia, consider exchange transfusion.

Admission Criteria

Admit to ICU if symptomatic or MetHgb >20%.

Pearls and Pitfalls

- Infants are particularly susceptible because erythrocyte b5R activity (an enzyme that reduces physiologically produced MetHgb back to hemoglobin) is 50%–60% of the normal adult activity.
- Glucose-6-phosphate dehydrogenase deficiency (G6PD): Methemoglobinemia in these patients will not respond to methylene blue because reduction of MetHgb by methylene blue is dependent on NADPH produced by G6PD.
- Keep in mind that agents may have toxicities unrelated to methemoglobinemia, such as seizures due to lidocaine or benzocaine.
- If there is known exposure to a specific agent, consult the poison control center or a clinical toxicologist because toxicities of agents may confuse the picture. (For example, paraquat, a pesticide, causes pulmonary fibrosis, and patients with overdoses may present with hypoxia, shortness of breath, and cyanosis. Supplemental oxygen is contraindicated. Nitrates are vasodilators and may present with hypotension, exacerbating the toxicity of methemoglobinemia.)

References and Suggested Readings

1. Goldfrank L, Flomenbaum N, Lewin N, et al, eds. *Goldfrank's toxicologic emergencies,* ed 7, New York, 2002, McGraw-Hill, pp 1438-1449.
2. Goldman L, Ausiello D, eds. *Cecil textbook of medicine,* ed 22, Philadelphia, 2004, WB Saunders, pp 1039-1041.
3. Wright RO, Lewander WJ, Woolf AD: Methemoglobinemia: etiology, pharmacology, and clinical management, *Ann Emerg Med* 34(5):646-656, 1999.

Chapter 19

Rhabdomyolysis

STEPHANIE WITT

Overview

Rhabdomyolysis is a clinical syndrome caused by injury to skeletal muscle that results in the release of its contents into the circulation. The final common pathway, regardless of the etiology, is damage to sarcolemma with release of intracellular contents such as myoglobin, lactate dehydrogenase, creatine phosphokinase, potassium, and phosphorus.

Substances

The **leading causes** of rhabdomyolysis are ethanol, drugs, infections, trauma, and seizures.
- Ethanol
  - Most common cause, especially binge drinking
  - Obtundation results in immobilization with external compression of blood supply
  - Directly toxic to muscle cells, potentiated by starvation
- Cocaine
  - Excessive energy demands, direct toxicity
  - CK > 5–10 × normal

Other Drugs

Amphetamines
Amphotericin B
Antimalarials
Aspirin
Barbiturates
Caffeine
Clofibrate
Cocaine
Codeine
Colchicine
Corticosteroids

Cyclic antidepressants
Diuretics
Ecstasy
Epsilon aminocaproic
   acid
Heroin
Isoniazid
Laxatives
Licorice
LSD

Major tranquilizers
Narcotics
PCP
Peanut oil
Phenylpropanolamine
Succinylcholine
Theophylline
Zidovudine
HMG-CoA reductase
   inhibitors

Toxins

Carbon monoxide
Ethanol
Ethylene glycol
2,4-Dichlorophenoxyacetic
   acid

Hall disease
Hemlock
Isopropyl alcohol

Mercuric chloride
Snake or spider bite
Toluene

- Metabolic
  - Any drug or condition that leads to hypokalemia, hyponatremia, hypophosphatemia
- Malignant hyperthermia
- Neuroleptic malignant syndrome
- Hypothermia

Toxicity

Sodium-potassium ATPase pump maintains sodium concentration. A mismatch between energy supply and demand, a defect in energy use, or direct injury results in increased permeability of the muscle cell → increased sodium concentration impairs sodium-calcium exchange → increased calcium → disinhibition or increased activity of proteolytic enzymes, which then cause damage to the cell.

Clinical Presentation

- 50% of patients complain of myalgia or muscle weakness.
- Only 4%–15% have the "classic" description of muscle weakness, tenderness, or swelling with discoloration of overlying skin.

Complications

- Acute renal failure
- Electrolyte abnormalities
  - Hyperkalemia
  - Hyperphosphatemia
  - Hypercalcemia (late in course) (patients with this also experience acute renal failure)
  - Hypocalcemia (early in course)
  - Hyperuricemia
- Hypoalbuminemia
- Compartment syndrome
- Disseminated intravascular coagulation (DIC)
- Respiratory insufficiency
- Hepatic insufficiency
- Peripheral neuropathy

Laboratory Evaluation

- Creatine phosphokinase (CPK) $\geq 5 \times$ normal
- Urine dipstick is positive for blood, but no red blood cells (RBCs) are seen microscopically.
- Consider CBC and DIC screen (PT, PTT, fibrin split products, fibrinogen), ABG, electrolytes, calcium, phosphorus, BUN, Cr.
- Blood myoglobin measurement is unreliable because of its short half-life; it peaks within 1–3 hr and disappears within 6 hr.

Treatment

- Hydration: IV crystalloid bolus for correction of fluid deficit, then infuse at 2.5 mL/kg/hr (or 1.5–2 × maintenance rate)
- Maintain urine output ≥ 2 mL/kg/hr or 200–300 mL/hr.
- For rhabdomyolysis resistant to hydration:
  - Mannitol (20%) 1 g/kg IV over 30 min or 25 g IV initially followed by 5 g/hr IV

- Consider only after appropriate volume replacement.
- Avoid in anuria. May carefully consider its use in early acute renal failure to convert oliguric renal failure to nonoliguric renal failure.
- Sodium bicarbonate 1 mEq/kg IV bolus or 100 mEq added to D_5W at 250 mL/hr for 4 hr
  - Maintain urine pH ≥ 6.5 to prevent acute renal failure (ARF).
  - Can exacerbate hypocalcemia
  - Prevents myoglobin dissociation into ferrihemate, which is toxic to the renal tubule
- Furosemide 20 mg IV (may require 40–200 mg IV). Caution: loop diuretics can acidify the urine.
- Hemodialysis

Special Considerations

- Hypocalcemia
  - No treatment required
  - Calcium only for hyperkalemia-induced cardiotoxicity or profound signs and symptoms of hypocalcemia
- Hypercalcemia
  - Frequently symptomatic
  - Normally responds to saline diuresis and furosemide
- Hyperphosphatemia
  - If ≥ 7 mg/dL, treat with oral phosphate binders.
- Hypophosphatemia
  - Treat if level ≤ 1 mg/dL.
- Hyperkalemia
  - Usually most severe in first 12–36 hr
  - Calcium, bicarbonate, insulin/glucose therapy, Kayexalate, dialysis

Admission Criteria

- Altered mental status
- Acute renal failure
- Significant toxicity from drug or toxin

Pearls and Pitfalls

- Ethanol is the most common cause of rhabdomyolysis.
- Hyperkalemia is most elevated in the first 12–36 hours.
- Maintaining a urine pH ≥ 6.5 may help prevent ARF.
- Consider rhabdomyolysis when there is positive blood on urine dip and no RBCs on microscopic exam.
- Myoglobinuric renal failure is the most commonly seen medical complication of PCP intoxication.

References and Suggested Readings

1. Goldfrank L, Flomenbaum N, Lewin N, et al, eds: *Goldfrank's toxicologic emergencies,* ed 7, 2002, Appleton and Lange, p 524.
2. Marx J, Hockberger R, Walls R: *Rosen's emergency medicine: concepts and clinical practice,* ed 5, St Louis, 2002, Mosby, pp 1762-1770.
3. Tintinalli J, Kelen G, Stapczynski J: *Emergency medicine: a comprehensive study guide,* ed 5, 2000, McGraw-Hill, pp 1841-1845.
4. Vanholder R, Sever M, Erek E, et al: Rhabdomyolysis, *J Am Soc Nephrol* 11:1553–1561, 2000.
5. Visweswaran P, Guntupalli J: Environmental emergencies: rhabdomyolysis, *Crit Care Clin* 15:415-428, 1999.

Chapter 20

Prolonged QT/QRS

Stephanie Witt

■ Overview

Drugs causing dysrhythmias or cardiac conduction abnormalities alter function of the myocardial cell membrane. The QRS complex reflects depolarization of ventricular myocardium. The QT interval reflects duration of depolarization and repolarization of ventricular myocardium. Inhibition of any of the sodium, calcium, or potassium channels involved in myocardial cell function will be reflected in QRS and/or QT interval abnormalities. Inhibition of fast sodium channels in phase 0 of the cardiac action potential causes prolonged depolarization, reflected by a prolonged QRS. Inhibition of potassium channels causes delayed repolarization, reflected by a prolonged QT interval.

■ Substances

Widened QRS/QTc	
β-blockers	Cyclic antidepressants
Calcium antagonists	Diphenhydramine
Class IA antidysrhythmics	Phenothiazines (especially thioridazine)
Class IC antidysrhythmics	Propoxyphene

- Class IA antidysrhythmics (Procainamide, Disopyramide, Quinidine [PDQ])
  - Depress rapid action potential upstroke
  - Decrease conduction velocity by sodium channel blockade
  - Prolong repolarization by potassium channel blockade
- Class IC (flecainide, moricizine, propafenone)
  - Depress rapid action potential upstroke
  - Decrease conduction velocity by sodium channel blockade
- Cyclic antidepressants have a quinidine-like effect
- Diphenhydramine in massive overdoses

Prolonged QT

Arsenic	Droperidol	Organophosphates
Atypical antipsychotics	Erythromycin	Phenothiazines*
Citalopram	Fluorides	Propoxyphene
Clarithromycin	Haloperidol	Scorpion or spider bite
Class Ia antidysrhythmics	Hypo Mg, K, Ca	Tamoxifen
Class III antidysrhythmics	Lithium	TMP-SMX
Contrast injection	Octreotide	Tricyclic antidepressants

The major phenothiazine culprits include thioridazine and thiothixene.

Toxicity

- Presence of prolonged QRS or QT → high risk of developing significant dysrhythmias
- Factors that contribute to development of dysrhythmias (e.g., torsades de pointes) include hypokalemia, hypomagnesemia, hypocalcemia, bradycardia, ischemia, and tissue hypoxia.
- Acquired prolonged QT (e.g., drug-induced) = "pause dependent" because torsades de pointes generally occurs at slow heart rates or in response to short-long-short RR interval sequences.
- Torsades de pointes is characterized by prolonged ventricular repolarization with QT intervals generally exceeding 500 ms. The abnormal repolarization may be apparent only on the beat prior to the onset of torsades de pointes (i.e., following a premature ventricular contraction).
- Initiation of torsades de pointes: PVC closely coupled with a normal QRS, then followed by a pause. The next sinus beat is closely coupled with a PVC, which is the first beat of torsades de pointes

Clinical Presentation

- QT prolongation with torsades de pointes is usually seen within 7 days of starting or altering drug therapy.
- Phenothiazines: Effects seen within 1–2 days of starting therapy, within 4–5 days maximum
- Delayed episodes (months) due to additive effect on ventricular repolarization (e.g., electrolyte abnormality or addition of another drug known to cause prolonged QT or torsades de pointes).
- **Torsades de pointes**
  - May present with syncope, but generally self-limited
  - Ventricular rate > 200 beats per minute (bpm)
  - QRS with undulating axis, shifting polarity about baseline because of numerous simultaneous ventricular tachycardia reentry foci competing to depolarize the ventricle
  - May also be caused by Class III agents (sotalol and amiodarone) and pentamidine; effects may persist for weeks after discontinuation.
  - Often short episodes (< 90 sec)
  - If unstable (hypotension, ischemia, heart failure), cardioversion is indicated (often ineffective) followed by lidocaine (also often ineffective)

Laboratory Evaluation

- EKG
- Electrolytes, including magnesium
- Chest radiograph
- **QT interval calculations**
  - QT interval (QTc <0.44 sec)
  - Bazett's formula: $QTc = (QT) \div (\sqrt{RR} \text{ [in sec]})$
  - "Poor man's guide" to upper limits of QT:
    - For HR of 70 bpm: QT < 0.40 sec
    - For every 10 bpm increase above 70, subtract 0.02 sec.
    - For every 10 bpm decrease below 70, add 0.02 sec.
  - Example:
    - QT <0.38 @ 80 bpm
    - QT <0.42 @ 60 bpm

Treatment

General

- ABCs, decontamination
- Correct metabolic abnormalities that may be further exacerbating toxicity.

- Supportive measures (oxygen, ECG monitoring)
- Treat dysrhythmias per ACLS protocol; **avoid** Class IA and Class IC agents.

Specific

- Sodium bicarbonate 1 mEq/kg
- Start infusion with 3 amps (150 mEq) in 850 mL D_5W at 200 mL/hr.
- ABG q 2 hours: Keep serum pH between 7.5 and 7.55.
- May stop bicarbonate when QRS < 100 ms, then check EKG after 6 hr.

Special Considerations

Torsades de Pointes

- Presume prolonged QRS/QT and subsequent dysrhythmia to be due to quinidine-like activity of cyclic antidepressant, phenothiazine, chloroquine, or antidysrhythmics. Treat with bicarbonate, then Class IB agent (lidocaine) for persistent dysrhythmia.
- Correct metabolic/electrolyte abnormalities.
- Magnesium 2 to 6 mg IV over 10 to 40 min (watch for changes in rhythm, respirations, reflexes, or blood pressure)
  - Causes calcium channel blockade and prevents calcium influx
- Lidocaine 1.5 mg/kg IV
- Isoproterenol infusion
- Overdrive pacing

Cyclic Antidepressants

See Chapter 3.

- Indication for specific treatment
- Widening of QRS
- QRS duration >100 ms in limb leads prognostic of seizures
- QRS duration >160 ms associated with cardiac dysrhythmias
- Rightward deviation of the terminal 40 ms QRS axis (R >3 mm in aVR)
- R wave in aVR >3 mm predictive of seizures or dysrhythmias
- R:S ratio >0.7 in aVR

Specific

- Sodium bicarbonate 1 mEq/kg
  - Start infusion with 3 amps (150 mEq) in 850 mL D_5W at 200 mL/hr.
- ABG q 2 hours: Keep serum pH between 7.5 and 7.55.
- May stop bicarbonate when QRS <100 ms, then check EKG after 6 hr.

Admission Criteria

- Patients presenting with ventricular dysrhythmias
- Patients with QTc of 500 or greater
- Bradycardia, hypotension, or conduction defects (i.e., second- and third-degree A-V blocks)

Pearls and Pitfalls

- Torsades de pointes is more likely when the QTc >500 ms.
- Torsades de pointes typically results when drugs inhibit potassium efflux during phase 3 of the action potential.
- Cyclic antidepressants have a quinidine-like effect (i.e., Na-channel blockade).
- QTc prolongation can be seen within 7 days of starting or altering a medication.
- Sodium bicarbonate or hypertonic saline may be helpful in treating drug toxicity leading to wide QRS.
- Amitriptyline may respond to sodium bicarbonate to a greater degree than to hypertonic saline.

References and Suggested Readings

1. Ellenhorn M, Schonwald S, Ordog G, et al, eds: *Ellenhorn's medical toxicology: Diagnosis and treatment of human poisoning,* ed 2, Baltimore, 1997, Williams & Wilkins, p 27.
2. Flinders DC, Roberts SD: Ventricular arrhythmias, *Prim Care* 27(3):709-724, 2000.
3. Goldfrank L, Flomenbaum N, Lewin N, et al, eds. *Goldfrank's toxicologic emergencies,* ed 6, Connecticut, 1998, Appleton and Lange, pp 116-117, 363-368.
4. Marx J, Hockberger R, Walls R: *Rosen's emergency medicine: concepts and clinical practice,* ed 5, St Louis, 2002, Mosby, pp 1095-1096.
5. Drugs that Prolong the Qt Interval and/or Induce Torsades de Pointes Ventricular Arrhythmia. http://torsades.org/medical-pros/drug-lists/drug-lists.htm. The University of Arizona Center for Education and Research on Therapeutics Arizona Health Sciences Center, Tucson, Arizona. Last updated Jun 14, 2006.

Chapter 21

Toxin-Induced Seizures

STEPHANIE WITT

Overview

Most seizures caused by drugs are generalized tonic-clonic seizures. Depending on the degree of toxicity, seizures may be isolated, recurrent, or continuous. Seizures can be a terminal event in almost any drug exposure.

Substances

There are many causes of toxin-induced seizures, but the most common causes are "WITH LA COPS." (See Section 3, "Mnemonics.")

Remember: WITH LA COPS	
W	Withdrawal (ethanol, benzodiazepine, GHB, Wellbutrin)
I	Isoniazid, Inderal, insulin, industrial acids, inhalants (anoxia)
T	Theophylline, TCA, Tramadol
H	Hypoglycemics, Haldol (lowers seizure threshold), hemlock, hydrazines
L	Lithium, lidocaine (local anesthetics), lead, lindane
A	Anticholinergics, anticonvulsants, antibiotics (quinolones, imipenem, dapsone)
C	Cocaine, camphor, cyanide, carbon monoxide, cholinergics
O	Organophosphates
P	PCP, phenylpropanolamine, propoxyphene (and meperidine)
S	Sympathomimetics, salicylates, strychnine, SSRI (Prozac, Celexa)

See Box 21-1 for a more comprehensive list of substances.

Toxicity

- Pathophysiology of seizures is dependent on the characteristics of the drug or toxin.
  - Direct CNS stimulation is caused by drugs such as methamphetamines and cocaine.
  - Sympathomimetics affect sodium channels and abruptly decrease seizure threshold.

BOX 21-1 ■ DRUG- OR TOXIN-INDUCED SEIZURES

Non-Prescription	Prescription	Psychotropic	Alcohols or Drugs	Botanical
Antihistamines	Antihistamines	Antiemetics	Amphe-tamines	Gaiega
Caffeine	Carbamazepine	Barbiturates	Cocaine	Jimson-weed
Ephedrine	Chloroquine	Benzos	Disulfiram	Lobelia
Mefenamic	Clonidine	Cyclic	Ethanol	Mandrake
Phenylbutazone	Digoxin	antidepressants	Ethylene	Mistletoe
Propanolamine	Ergotamines	Lithium	glycol	Nicotine
Salicylates	General	MAO-I	MDMA	Passion
	anesthetic	Methyl-phenidate	Methanol	flower
	Imipenem	Neuroleptics	Phen-cyclidine	Periwinkle
	Isoniazid	Opioids		Pokeweed
	Lidocaine	(propoxyphene,		Rhodo-dendron
	Methotrexate	meperidine)		Worm-wood
	Phenytoin			
	Quinine			
	Sulfonylureas			
	Theophylline			

Heavy metals	Household toxins	Pesticides	Occupational	Animals
Arsenic	Benzalkonium	Diquat/	Carbon	Marine
Copper	chloride	paraquat	disulfide	animals
Lead	Boric acid	Organochlo-rines	Carbon	(Gymnothorax,
Manganese	Camphor	(lindane)	monoxide	saxitoxin
Nickel	Fluoride	Organo-phosphates	Cyanide	[shellfish])
	Hexachloro-phene	Rodenticides	Hydrocarbons	Pit viper
	Phenol	(strychnine)	Hydrogen	Scorpion
			sulphide	Tick bite
			Methyl bromide	*(Rickettsia)*
			Toxic inhalants	

Adapted from Goldfrank LR, Flomenbaum N, Lewin N, et al, eds: Goldfrank's toxicologic emergencies, *ed 6, New Haven 1998, Appleton & Lange, p 323.*

- γ-Aminobutyric acid (GABA) and glycine are inhibitory neurotransmitters. Interference with normal neurotransmission causes CNS disinhibition, such as in isoniazid-induced seizures.
- A toxin can have more than one mechanism of stimulation. For example, cocaine causes direct CNS stimulation, lowers seizure threshold, and causes cardiac toxicity, which leads to hypoxemia, another contributing factor in seizures.

Clinical Presentation

Seizure, of course.

Laboratory Evaluation

- Metabolic screening for electrolyte disorders, hypoglycemia, uremia
- CBC with platelets
- INR, PTT (if extracorporeal drug removal becomes necessary)
- Urine toxicology screen
- Urine pregnancy test
- Acetaminophen level if ingestion suspected
- CK if multiple or protracted seizures (rhabdomyolysis)
- Lab testing specific to a suspected ingestion (e.g., theophylline level)
- Consider other causes of seizure such as infection.
- Remember principles of first-time seizure evaluation (i.e., head CT, liver enzymes, ammonia).

Treatment

- ABCs, ensure secure airway
- Thiamine 100 mg IV and magnesium 1–2 g IV in alcoholic patients
- Dextrose (50 mL [1 amp] of D_{50} IV in adults, 2–4 mL/kg of D_{25} in children) if hypoglycemic
- Lorazepam 0.1 mg/kg (adults)
  - 0.05–0.1 mg/kg IV (children: 4 mg maximal single dose)
  - Longer duration of action than diazepam
- **or** diazepam 5–10 mg IV q 5 min up to 20 mg (adults)
  - 0.3 mg/kg (children: 10 mg maximal single dose)
  - Faster onset than lorazepam
- Fosphenytoin 20 mgPE/kg IV (adults and children): faster onset and fewer side effects than phenytoin but more expensive

- **or** phenytoin 20 mg/kg IV
- Phenobarbital 20 mg/kg IV (adults and children), may repeat 5–10 mg/kg IV
- General anesthesia with midazolam (0.2 mg/kg, then 0.75–10 μg/kg/min), or propofol (1–2 mg/kg, then 1–15 mg/kg/hr), or pentobarbital (10–15 mg/kg over 1 hr, then 0.5–1.0 mg/kg/hr)
- If necessary, consider short-term paralysis to control muscle contractions and facilitate treatment. Remember that abnormal neuronal activity will continue, which leads to brain damage if it is not controlled.
- Once seizures are controlled, consider appropriate gut decontamination (e.g., charcoal).

Special Considerations

Alcohol Withdrawal

- 6–48 hr after cessation or precipitous decline of alcohol use
- Generalized seizure, postictal period <30 min
- **Treatment**
  - D_5NS, thiamine, magnesium, 2 IVs
  - Diazepam 2–4 mg/min IV, up to 20 mg in first IV, start drip if seizures persist
  - Phenytoin 13–20 mg/kg IV in second IV
  - Phenobarbital if unable to use phenytoin

Isoniazid (INH)

- Seizures occur with doses ≥20 mg/kg.
  - Lower doses are required to induce seizures in people with underlying seizure disorder.
- Causes GABA deficiency (inhibitory neurotransmitter) by binding pyridoxine, which is necessary for GABA production
- Overdose can be associated with seizures refractory to conventional therapy, metabolic acidosis, persistent coma
- Usually symptomatic within 30–45 min postingestion, seizures within 2 hr
- Usually generalized tonic-clonic seizure, but may be focal
- Often develops into status epilepticus refractory to anticonvulsants
- **Treatment**
  - Pyridoxine synergistic with benzodiazepine for seizure control
    - Pyridoxine 1 g IV per 1 g INH ingested to maximum of 5 g, give 1 g every 2–3 min (Replenishing pyridox-

ine allows the body to produce GABA, which is an essential inhibitory neurotransmitter.)
- If amount ingested is unknown: Pyridoxine 5 g IV (adult), 70 mg/kg (child) up to maximum 5 g
- May repeat dose if seizures recur
- If seizures are controlled before full amount is given, mix remainder with D_5W and infuse slowly.
- Phenytoin is ineffective.
- Diazepam 5–10 mg IV at rate of 5 mg/min (repeat q 10–15 min up to 30 mg)
  - Child: 0.3–0.5 mg/kg IV q 15–30 min up to 10 mg maximum
  - 0.5 mg/kg PR if IV cannot be established
- Lorazepam 0.1 mg/kg IV q 5–7 min (maximum 8 mg adults, 4 mg child)
- Activated charcoal once seizures are controlled
- IV Fluids: D_5NS
- Bicarbonate for acidosis not responsive to fluids, pyridoxine, and diazepam

Cocaine

- Seizures usually occur within 90 min (but up to 12 hr) of cocaine use.
- Usually generalized seizure
- Focal seizures are more likely in the patient with a history of seizure disorder, but intracranial hemorrhage or infarction must be considered.
- **Treatment:** Benzodiazepines

Strychnine

- Rodenticides in the form of crystal or white powder, absorbed through GI tract or nasal mucosa, still sold in tonics and cathartic pills in health food stores
- Signs and symptoms begin within 15–20 min of ingestion.
- Competitive antagonism of inhibitory neurotransmitter **glycine** at postsynaptic spinal cord motor neuron
- Painful "seizures": muscle twitching, extensor spasm, opisthotonos, trismus, or facial grimacing (*risus sardonicus*)
- Conscious between episodes
- **Treatment**
  - Activated charcoal
  - If symptomatic: quiet environment, benzodiazepine, pain medicine to avoid any stimulation that may precipitate opisthotonos or convulsions

- Diazepam 0.1–0.5 mg/kg followed by barbiturate such as pentobarbital
- If the above are ineffective, general anesthesia/intubation with nondepolarizing neuromuscular blockade (e.g., vecuronium) should be considered.

Tricyclic Antidepressants (TCAs)

- EKG: QRS >100 ms, R ≥3 mm in aVR is predictive of seizure development.
- **Treatment**
  - Benzodiazepines are the agent of choice. Consider midazolam if refractory to other benzos.
  - Propofol (2.5 mg/kg load, then 0.2 mg/kg/min) or phenobarbital for refractory seizures
  - **Do not use phenytoin if suspect TCA overdose** because it has similar antiarrhythmic properties as TCA → exacerbate cardiac abnormalities.
  - Sodium bicarbonate is useful only for treating the cardiotoxic effects of TCAs (by partially reversing the fast sodium channel blockade caused by the drug). It will not work for treatment of TCA-induced seizures.

Theophylline

- Theophylline antagonizes the depressant effect of adenosine on the cerebral cortex and increases tissue levels of cyclic AMP, a potentially epileptogenic substance.
- Seizures may be an initial sign of toxicity in chronic overmedication.
- Major toxicity (i.e., seizures, arrhythmias) are more common with *chronic intoxication,* despite lower theophylline levels compared with acute ingestion, and may occur at therapeutic or mildly toxic levels.
- Single toxic dose >10 mg/kg
- Lab: Theophylline levels every 2 hr until decline is noted in 2 successive levels, then levels every 4–6 hr until values are less than 20 μg/mL
- **Treatment**
  - May not respond to usual treatment (diazepam, phenytoin)
  - General anesthesia (e.g., with thiopental) if seizures are continuous and last more than 1 hr in adults or 30 min in children
  - Hemoperfusion is the extracorporeal elimination method of choice for theophylline elimination. Indications for charcoal hemoperfusion include theophylline level

>90 μg/mL at any time or theophylline level >40 μg/mL in association with seizures, hypotension unresponsive to fluid resuscitation, ventricular dysrhythmias, or protracted vomiting that does not respond to antiemetics.
- Hemodialysis is a reasonable alternative if hemoperfusion is not available.

Admission Criteria

- Admission or discharge after short-term observation is based on the physician's judgment.
- In general, patients with toxicity severe enough to cause seizures merit admission for further observation and monitoring of other adverse effects (e.g., cardiac toxicity) that may be associated with the drug.

Pearls and Pitfalls

- In general, a benzodiazepine (commonly either diazepam or lorazepam) is the first-line agent in seizure management.
- Benzodiazepines are often titrated to effect. "Maximal" doses listed are not absolute. However, if dosing reaches the "maximal" levels, one must consider airway protection (i.e., intubation).
- Phenytoin is often ineffective in alcohol withdrawal seizures.
- Always remember that if a patient is paralyzed and intubated, EEG monitoring is the only way to monitor for persistent seizure activity until the paralysis resolves.

References and Suggested Readings

1. Ellenhorn MJ, Schonwald S, Ordog G, et al, eds: *Ellenhorn's medical toxicology,* ed 2, Baltimore, 1997, Williams & Wilkins, pp 113-114, 240-241, 370, 627-628, 831-834, 1144.
2. Goldfrank LR, Flomenbaum N, Lewin N, et al, eds: *Goldfrank's toxicologic emergencies,* ed 6, Hartford, 1998, Appleton & Lange, pp 323, 730-731, 1464-1465.
3. Hanhan U, Fiallos M: Pediatric critical care: a new millenium: status epilepticus, *Pediatr Clin North Am* 48:683-694, 2001.
4. Liebelt E, Francis P, Woolf A: ECG lead aVR versus QRS interval in predicting seizures and arrhythmias in acute tricyclic antidepressant toxicity, *Ann Emerg Med* 26:195-201, 1995.
5. Tintinalli J, Kelen G, Stapcznski J: *Emergency medicine: a comprehensive study guide,* ed 5, New York, 2000, McGraw-Hill, pp 1463-1471.

Chapter 22

Metabolic Acidosis with Anion Gap

STEPHANIE WITT

■ Overview

Anion gap = unmeasured anions − unmeasured cations = $Na^+ - (Cl^- + HCO_3^-)$

The preceding equation reflects the difference between amount of anions and cations in serum. Normal anion gap is due to anions such as albumin, phosphate, sulfate, and organic acids. If the anion gap is elevated, there is either an increase in the unmeasured anions or a decrease in the number of cations. An anion gap >20 mmol/L signifies metabolic acidosis, regardless of pH or serum bicarbonate concentration. The patient with a higher anion gap tends to have increased severity of illness, although the absence of anion gap does not exclude significant illness.

▥ Causes

> ### Remember: **MUDPILE CATS.**
>
> | | |
> |---|---|
> | **M** | Methanol, metformin |
> | **U** | Uremia |
> | **D** | Diabetic ketoacidosis |
> | **P** | Paraldehyde, phenformin |
> | **I** | Iron, isoniazid, ibuprofen, idiopathic |
> | **L** | Lithium, lactate |
> | **E** | Ethylene glycol, ethanol |
> | **C** | Carbon monoxide, cyanide, caffeine |
> | **A** | Alcoholic ketoacidosis |
> | **T** | Toluene, theophylline |
> | **S** | Salicylates, hydrogen sulfide, strychnine, sympathomimetic amines, starvation ketoacidosis |

▥ Toxicity

Toxicity depends on the cause.

▥ Clinical Presentation

Clinical presentation may help with etiology, as follows:
- No GI symptoms → not iron toxicity
- No seizures → not isoniazid toxicity
- Visual complaints or abnormal fundoscopic exam ("stepping out into a snowstorm" [e.g., cloudy, indistinct vision, dense central scotoma]) → methanol, ethylene glycol
- Characteristic odor = paraldehyde
- Increased respiratory rate and diaphoresis could be salicylate toxicity or diabetic ketoacidosis (DKA).

▥ Laboratory Evaluation

- Chem-8: BUN, creatinine, hyperglycemia, anion gap
- Urinalysis for:
  - Glucose and ketones
  - Calcium oxalate crystals (ethylene glycol)
  - Fluorescence with Wood's lamp (ethylene glycol)

- If absent, does not rule out ethylene glycol
- Ferric chloride (see Chapter 1, "Salicylates")
- ABG: pH, respiratory processes/compensation
  - Prediction of degree of respiratory compensation in acute metabolic acidosis:

$$pCO_2 = 1.5(HCO_3^-) + 8 \pm 2$$

  - If pure compensated metabolic acidosis: pCO_2 = last 2 digits of pH (e.g., pH 7.26 → pCO_2 = 26 if pure compensated metabolic acidosis)
  - If pCO_2 does not correspond with either of the above prediction rules, consider any respiratory processes that are occurring.
- Lactate level: Can be considered lactic acidosis if lactate can account for fall in serum bicarbonate
  - Anion gap may not be elevated in 50% of patients with moderate lactic acidosis and in 80% of patients with mild lactic acidosis.
  - Lactate level >2.5 mmol/L is abnormal.
  - Increasing lactate levels correspond to increasing mortality. A patient with a lactate level > 10 mmol/L can have a mortality rate approaching 100%.
  - If labs do not suggest etiology: usually toxic alcohol ingestion
- Also consider: starvation alcoholic ketoacidosis (preceded by prolonged, massive ingestion of ethanol, abruptly terminated by abdominal pain and vomiting with minimal ketonuria and no glucosuria), multifactorial etiology involving small amounts of lactate and other ions.
- Osmolal gap (see Chapter 23) suggests toxic alcohol ingestion.

▌ Treatment

- Hydration, dextrose, thiamine → if resolution → likely ketoacidosis or lactic acidosis
- If a specific cause is found, treat specifically (e.g., DKA = fluids, insulin/glucose; uremia = dialysis; isoniazid = Vitamin B_6 and gut decontamination).

Special Considerations

- Metabolic acidosis in an infant: Consider inborn errors of metabolism.
  - The most frequent cause of metabolic acidosis in this age group is probably lactic acidosis.
- Children and especially toddlers are susceptible to ingesting many agents causing elevated anion gap metabolic acidosis: antifreeze, aspirin, iron (some preparations resemble candy), and ethanol. In addition, Münchausen's syndrome should be considered when there are inconsistencies or suspicions in this history.

Admission Criteria

- Admission depends on clinical presentation and diagnosis.
- The patient in obviously serious condition should be admitted to ICU.

Pearls and Pitfalls

- Acronyms and mnemonics do not list **all** etiologies of metabolic acidosis.
- Never forget to obtain a complete history and physical, which will guide your workup and management.
- Anion gap >20 mmol/L = metabolic acidosis, regardless of pH or serum bicarbonate concentration.
- High lactate of >10 mmol/L is associated with nearly 100% mortality.

References and Suggested Readings

1. Ellenhorn M, Schonwald S, Ordog G, et al, eds: *Ellenhorn's medical toxicology: diagnosis and treatment of human poisoning*, ed 2, Baltimore, 1997, Williams & Wilkins, pp 48-49, 119-123.
2. Goldfrank L, Flomenbaum N, Lewin N, et al, eds: *Goldfrank's toxicologic emergencies*, ed 6, Newport, 1998, Appleton & Lange, pp 245-247.
3. Wilson WC: Clinical approach to acid-base analysis: importance of the anion gap, *Anesthesiol Clin North Am* 19:907-912, 2001.

Chapter 23

Osmolal Gap

STEPHANIE WITT

Overview

The difference between measured osmolality and calculated osmolality is the osmolal gap.

$$\text{Calculated (mOsm)} = 2\,Na^+\,(mEq/L) + \text{glucose (mg/dL)}/18 + \text{BUN (mg/dL)}/2.8 + \text{ethanol (mg/dL)}/4.6$$

The normal osmolal gap in children is in the range of -14 to $+10\,mOsm/L$ and -2 to $10\,mOsm/L$ in the adult population. A large gap suggests toxic alcohol ingestion. To estimate the contribution of a toxic alcohol, use the following conversion factors:

Ethylene glycol = 6.2
Methanol = 3.2
Ethanol = 4.6

Alcoholic ketoacidosis, lactic acidosis, renal failure, and shock are all associated with elevated osmolal gap. **Small or negative osmolal gaps will not exclude toxic alcohol ingestion** (e.g., $1\,mEq/L$ error in Na^+ affects gap by $2\,mOsm$; ethylene glycol level of $50\,mg/dL$ only contributes $7.8\,mOsm/L$). If there is an osmolal gap and anion gap but no ethanol is present, this is strong evidence of poisoning by methanol or ethylene glycol. The longer the interval between time of ingestion and measuring of the osmols, the lower the gap.

Substances

> **Remember: ME DIE (if I drink this stuff).**
>
> M   Methanol
> E   Ethanol, ether
> D   Diuretics (mannitol, sorbitol, glycerine), dyes
> I   Isopropyl alcohol
> E   Ethylene glycol

Toxicity

Toxicity is cause specific.

Clinical Presentation

Clinical presentation is cause specific.

Laboratory Evaluation

- Toxicology screen for volatile alcohols
- Chemistry panel with electrolytes, BUN, Cr, glucose, calcium, anion gap
- Depending on presentation: chest radiograph, EKG, CT scan of head

Treatment

Treatment is cause specific. Treatment of methanol or ethylene glycol toxicity is either ethanol infusion or fomepizole (4-methylpyrazole) infusion; either substance competitively inhibits alcohol dehydrogenase, the enzyme that converts methanol and ethylene glycol to their toxic metabolites. Hemodialysis may also be considered.

Special Considerations

Remember, the range for osmolal gap in children is different than that in adults, –14 to 10 mOsm/L in children compared with –2 to 10 mOsm/L in adults.

Disposition

Admit all patients who are ill, have metabolic abnormalities, altered mental status, or who may require dialysis. Intentional ingestions will also require psychiatric evaluation.

Pearls and Pitfalls

- Think about obtaining measured osmolarity in patients with altered mental status.
- The longer the interval between time of ingestion and measuring of the osmols, the lower the gap.
- Small or negative osmolal gaps will not exclude toxic alcohol ingestion.
- Other causes include mannitol, acetone, and dimethyl sulfoxide (DMSO).
- The toxic acids generated from the toxic alcohols (EG and methanol) do not contribute to the osmolal gap.

References and Suggested Readings

1. Ellenhorn M, Schonwald S, Ordog G, et al, eds: *Ellenhorn's medical toxicology,* ed 2, Baltimore, 1997, Williams & Wilkins, pp 49-50.
2. Goldfrank L, Flomenbaum N, Lewin, N, et al, eds: *Goldfrank's toxicologic emergencies,* ed 6, Stamford, 1998, Appleton & Lange, pp 248-249.
3. Keyes DC: Toxicity, ethylene glycol. http://www.emedicine.com/emerg/topic177.htm Accessed Feb 1, 2005.
4. McQuillen KK, Anderson AC: Osmol gaps in the pediatric population, *Acad Emerg Med* 6:27-30, 1999.
5. Mycyk MB, Acks SE: A visual schematic for clarifying the temporal relationship between the anion and osmol gaps in toxic alcohol poisoning, *Am J Emerg Med* 21:333-335, 2003.

Chapter 24

Over-Anticoagulation

Stephanie Witt

Overview

Warfarin inhibits activation of vitamin K, which is necessary for production of coagulation factors II, VII, IX, and X. Only free warfarin is active; drugs that alter binding affect anticoagulation. Warfarin is a CYP 1A2 enzyme substrate (minor); CYP2C8, 2C9, 2C18, 2C19, and 3A4 enzyme substrate; and CYP2C9 enzyme inhibitor. Therefore, any drug that affects (either induces or inhibits) these enzyme systems may alter coagulation status.

Substances

Other herbals that have not been studied but have coumarin-like substances that may interact with warfarin include horse chestnut, red clover, sweet clover, and sweet woodruff.

Anticoagulant Drug Overdose/Ingestion	
Hydroxycourmarin	Indanedione
Brodifacoum	Chlorphacinone
Bromadiolone	Diphacinone
Coumachlor	Pindone
Fumarin	Valone
Warfarin	

Substances with Clinically Significant Drug Interactions*

Antimicrobials	Antituberculars	Analgesics	Others
Chloramphenicol	Isoniazid	Acetaminophen	Allopurinol
Ciprofloxacin	Rifampin	(large doses)	Boldo
Clarithromycin		ASA	Danshen
Erythromycin	**Antiarrhythmics**	Indomethacin	Diazoxide
Metronidazole	Amiodarone	Ketoprofen	Digibind
TMP-SMX	Propafenone	NSAIDs	Dipyridamole
Tetracycline		Phenylbutazone	Disulfiram
	Antihyperlipidemics	Tolmetin	Dong quai
H₂ blockers	Clofibrate	Salicylates	Fenugreek
Cimetidine	Gemfibrozil	Sulindac	Garlic
Omeprazole	Lovastatin		Ginkgo
Ranitidine			Papaya
	Antifungals		Tamoxifen
Anticonvulsants	Fluconazole		Vitamin E
Phenobarbital	Itraconazole		
Phenytoin	Miconazole		

Interactions resulting in increased PT/INR.

▮ Toxicity

In the early 1920s, livestock that were inadvertently fed moldy sweet clover hay developed hemorrhagic disorders. It was later found that the coumarin in sweet clover is oxidized to the anti-coagulant 4-bishydroxycoumarin by fungi in moldy sweet clover, which caused the bleeding.

- As mentioned above, warfarin inhibits activation of vitamin K, which is necessary for production of coagulation factors II, VII, IX, and X.
- The typical rodenticide contains small concentrations of anticoagulant (0.025% or 25 mg of warfarin per 100 g of product).
- The amount of warfarin required even in a child to have significant anticoagulation is far greater than what is ingested in a "taste" → single, unintentional ingestions pose little to no threat.
- Normally the patient with an acute warfarin overdose recovers in about 5 days (T½= 6–23 days), but the clinical effects secondary to the long half-life of the superwarfarins may persist for weeks to months.

- Superwarfarins are long-acting anticoagulants (e.g., difenacoum, brodifacoum, chlorophacinone).
  - Same mechanism of action as warfarin
  - High lipid solubility
  - Selective concentration in liver
  - 100× more potent than warfarin
  - Single, unintentional ingestion is unlikely to result in increased PT or INR.
  - Small, repeated ingestions can result in clinically significant coagulopathy.
  - Intentional overdose characterized by severe coagulopathy that lasts for weeks to months with consequential blood loss
  - Most common sites of bleeding: GI and GU
  - Based on the half-life of factor VII, a measurable effect on coagulation does not occur for 15–24 hr.
  - Bleeding is usually seen for 2–3 days postingestion or longer.

Clinical Presentation

- Typical manifestations of impaired coagulation
  - Anorexia, nausea, vomiting, diarrhea
  - Bruising, petechiae, persistent oozing from superficial injuries, skin necrosis
  - Hematuria
  - Hematochezia, melena, hemoptysis
  - Menorrhagia
- Rare but life-threatening complications such as neck hematoma with airway compromise, intracranial hemorrhage (typically lobar), pulmonary hemorrhage
- Purple toe syndrome
  - Rare complication
  - Purplish discoloration on plantar and axial surfaces of the toes
  - Occurs within 3–8 weeks of therapy initiation
  - Painful, tender, and fades with leg elevation. Blanching occurs with pressure.

Laboratory Evaluation

- CBC because abnormalities may include leukocytosis or anemia.
  - Platelets are usually normal.

- Bleeding time
- Prothrombin time with INR, activated partial thromboplastin time
- Rarely do coumarin anticoagulants cause elevation of liver enzymes.

▊ Treatment

- **Acute, unintentional ingestion:** Most patients are asymptomatic (usually children) with normal coagulation profile (PT, PTT, INR).
  - GI decontamination with activated charcoal if a large or unknown amount has been ingested and the patient arrives to the ED within 1 hr.
  - Nonintervention recommended because of the low risk of coagulopathy, which would occur over days.
  - PT becomes abnormal within 48 hr with superwarfarin. If it becomes abnormal → serial PT at 24 and 48 hr to identify patients at risk.
  - Do not give vitamin K prophylaxis: It will not be sufficient if coagulopathy does develop because coagulopathy will last for weeks; it delays detection of coagulopathy; and the gradual decline of coagulation factors prevents development of life-threatening anticoagulation in a single day.
- **Intentional ingestion**
  - GI decontamination (charcoal) may be effective if given within 1 hr postingestion.
  - Cholestyramine 12–16 g daily in divided doses (clears warfarin, interrupts enterohepatic circulation)
  - Admit for observation for onset of coagulopathy, PT once or twice daily.
  - If bleeding is evident – large bore IV, type and cross-match blood and fresh frozen plasma (FFP).
  - FFP: Initial treatment of choice for patients with active blood loss. Infuse as needed based on clinical symptoms and sequential PT/INR.
  - Vitamin K_1 for long-term PT control. May use parenteral 5–10 mg IV (IV or SQ). Usually SQ is preferred to IV due to anaphylactic concern. If IV is going to be used, it must be given over **at least** 30 min in adults or 1–5 mg IV in children initially (for 1 bolus or 1 day) and then switch to oral. Up to 50–100 mg per day may be required.
  - Half-life of vitamin K is short. If vitamin K is stopped, coagulopathy should reappear in 24–48 hr.

- Follow until coagulation studies are normal for several days after therapy has been stopped.
- Periodic coagulation factor analysis is an early clue to resolution.
- Intentional and large ingestions of pharmaceutical-grade anticoagulant → potential to produce coagulopathy and consequential bleeding.
- Treat similar to superwarfarins.
- See Table 24-1.
- In patients requiring chronic anticoagulation:
  - Observe if INR <5.0, no consequential bleeding, and patient is in a protected environment where trauma is unlikely (may require hospitalization).
- If INR significantly elevated or there is significant bleeding, give FFP periodically for partial and temporary reversal.
- If vitamin K_1 is given, complete reversal may occur and patient may be difficult to reanticoagulate.
- Use heparin if patient still needs anticoagulation but complete reversal of PT prolongation is desired or occurs with treatment.
- Patients not requiring chronic anticoagulation:
  - May treat with vitamin K_1 if PT is elevated.

▎ Special Considerations

Heparin

Bleeding occurs more commonly from appropriate administration of heparin rather than inappropriate high-dose administration.

Table 24-1 TREATMENT GUIDELINES FOR OVER-ANTICOAGULATION

INR	Treatment
<5	None
5.0–9.0	
No bleeding	None
Bleeding	Vitamin K_1 2.5 mg PO
>9.0	
No bleeding	Vitamin K_1 2.5–5 mg PO
Serious bleeding	Vitamin K_1 5–10 mg diluted in 100 mL D5W given IV slow (<1 mg/min); repeat dose q 12 hr
	FFP

FFP, Fresh frozen plasma.

- Accelerates binding of antithrombin III to thrombin, causing inhibition
- Duration of effect is short (1–3 days).
- Half-life is 60–90 min.
- Most reported cases involve unintentional poisoning.
- Management
  - No significant bleeding: Observation
    - **Monitor APTT serially in patients requiring anticoagulation.**
  - Significant bleeding: Replace blood loss.
    - Life-threatening hemorrhage: **Protamine** sulfate 1 mg/100 U of heparin, calculated based on dose of heparin administered and half-life of heparin
  - Protamine has many adverse effects. The worst is anaphylaxis, which occurs in about 0.2% of patients. However, the mortality rate is approximately 30%.
  - Hypotension (rate related and non–rate related)
  - Bradycardia
  - Thrombocytopenia
  - Give protamine over 15 min; monitor clotting parameters for 24 hr.
  - Hematology consultation

Low-Molecular-Weight (LMW) Heparins

- Targeted activity against factor X
- Greater bioavailability, longer half-life
- Management
  - Supportive
  - Newer (safer) experimental protamine variants are effective against LMW heparins.

Pregnancy

Pregnancy is usually a contraindication to the use of warfarin (category X) due to the association with birth defects known as *fetal warfarin syndrome.*

- Face hypoplasia
- Bone stippling of epiphysis
- Optic atrophy
- Mental retardation

Heparin is usually substituted for warfarin therapy in pregnant women.

Admission Criteria

Admit all patients with any of the following:

- Intracranial bleeding
- GI bleeding
- Other significant bleeding from GU or pulmonary systems or located in a potentially life-threatening area such as the neck
- Intentional overdose

Pearls and Pitfalls

- The term *warfarin* is derived from the patent holder (Wisconsin Area Research Foundation) and coum*arin*.
- Warfarin inhibits the **activation** of vitamin K.
- Superwarfarins are long-acting anticoagulants that are 100× more potent than coumarin.
- Beware of drug interactions that might increase anticoagulation.
- Unintentional ingestions of oral anticoagulants are rarely significant.

References and Suggested Readings

1. Atreja A, El-Sameed YA, Jneid H, et al: Elevated international normalized ratio in the ED: clinical course and physician adherence to the published recommendations, *Am J Emerg Med* 23:40-44, 2005.

2. *DRUG-REAX® System* [intranet database]. Greenwood Village, Colo: Thomson Micromedex, March 2004.

3. Ellenhorn M, Schonwald S, Ordog G, et al, eds: *Ellenhorn's medical toxicology: diagnosis and treatment of human poisoning*, ed 2, Baltimore, 1997, Williams & Wilkins, pp 452-463.

4. Goldfrank L, Flomenbaum N, Lewin N, et al, eds: *Goldfrank's toxicologic emergencies*, ed 6, Stamford; 1998, Appleton & Lange, pp 703-723.

5. Suchard JR, Curry SC. Oral Anticoagulants. In: Brent J, Wallace K, Burkhart K, et al, eds: *Critical care toxicology*, Philadelphia, 2005, Mosby, pp 695-700.

Chapter 25

Chemical Warfare (Primer)

STEPHANIE WITT

Overview

Chemical warfare is no longer a military threat per se. With increasing fears of terrorist attacks on civilian populations, clinicians need to be familiar with the agents that could potentially be used on civilians.

Agents typically used for chemical warfare are generally stored and transported as liquids. They can be deployed as liquid aerosols or vapors, leading to toxicity through skin, eyes, and respiratory tract exposure. At present, the possible use of these agents by terrorist groups is the subject of high vigilance, and many institutions organize preparedness exercises so that they are able to effectively and efficiently manage mass casualties due to these agents.

▓ Substances

Nerve agents

Sarin, soman, cyclosarin, tabun, VX

Vesicating or blistering agents

Sulfur mustard: also known as HD, which is a more purified or distilled
  form of sulfur mustard
Nitrogen mustards with potential warfare use: HN1, HN2, HN3
  (halogenated tertiary aliphatic amines that are colorless and odorless oily
  liquids)
Lewisite: an organic arsenical liquid that is colorless and oily with very little
  odor when purified. The synthesized chemical agent has a geranium-like
  odor and is a yellow to dark-brown liquid.

Choking agents or lung toxicants (chlorine, phosgene, diphosgene)

Chlorine: involved in more than 200 major accidental or unintentional
  releases per year; greenish-yellow gas
Phosgene: used in the dye industry but can be released when heating or
  burning chlorinate hydrocarbons

Cyanides (see Chapter 15)

Can be generated in fires in which plastic, wool, or silk are involved; also
  used in plastics and metals industries

Others (not discussed in this section)

Incapacitating agents (anticholinergics)
Lacrimating or riot control agents (pepper gas)
Vomiting agents (adamsite)

▓ Toxicity

Nerve Agents

These agents are similar to organophosphates and will phos-
phorylate and inactivate acetylcholinesterase. However, these
agents have a C-P bond not found in organophosphate pesticides, which is very resistant to hydrolysis.

- Acetylcholine accumulation → stimulation, then paralysis
  of cholinergic neurotransmission.
- Directly bind to nicotinic and muscarinic receptors
- Antagonize γ-aminobutyric acid (GABA) and stimulate
  glutamate *N*-methyl-D-aspartate (NMDA) receptors
- All are volatile liquids but are heavier than air, so they sink
  to low places.

- They rapidly penetrate skin and clothing.
- Fatality occurs rapidly regardless of the route of exposure.

Vesicating and Blistering Agents

- Cause blistering of exposed surface
- Rapid penetration of cells → formation of highly toxic intermediate → irreversible alkylation of DNA, RNA, and protein → disruption of cell function → cell death.
- Warm, moist tissues are more severely affected.
- Actively reproducing cells are most vulnerable (e.g., epithelial, hematopoietic).
- Deplete glutathione → inactivation of sulfhydryl-containing enzymes, loss of calcium homeostasis, lipid peroxidation, cell membrane breakdown, cell death.
- Oily liquid with mustard, onion, garlic, or horseradish odor → highly soluble in oils, fats, and organic solvents → quickly penetrate skin and most materials
- Mustard vapor (formed at high ambient temperatures) is the primary concern, but liquid is also very toxic.

Choking Agents

- Chlorine is a strong irritant, but in high concentrations it may be corrosive to mucous membranes if inhaled or ingested.
  - Acute injury to the lungs peaks in 12–24 hr.
  - Chlorine combines with tissue water to produce HCl, producing injury and reactive oxygen species.
  - Alveolar capillary congestion develops and leads to hypoxemia and hypercapnea. This is followed by atelectasis, emphysema, and respiratory and lactic acidosis.
  - Severe hypoxia and acidosis lead to cardiac arrest and death.
  - Is caustic to the eyes, skin, nose, throat, and mucous membranes
  - Exposures to various concentrations of chlorine gas are detailed in Table 25-1.
- Phosgene has the odor of freshly mown hay, grass, or green corn.
- Primarily a lower respiratory tract toxin. Low water solubility is one explanation for lack of upper respiratory tract irritant effects.
- When it contacts water, HCl is formed, leading to subsequent injury.
- Increases vascular permeability in the lung

Table 25-1 EFFECTS OF CHLORINE GAS CONCENTRATIONS

Chlorine Gas Concentrations	Effects
14 ppm for 30 min	Severe pulmonary damage
430 ppm or more for 30 min *or*	May be fatal
34–51 ppm for 60 min	May be fatal
1000 ppm	Fatal within a few breaths

Cyanides

See Chapter 15.

▌ Clinical Presentation

Nerve Agents

These agents cause muscarinic, nicotinic, and direct CNS toxicity.

- **Liquid:** symptoms 30 min to 18 hr after dermal exposure (Box 25-1)
- **Vapor:** symptoms within seconds to several minutes (Box 25-2)
- Other clinical signs and symptoms are shown in Box 25-3.

Vesicating and Blistering Agents

The clinical effects of these agents depend on the form in which it is distributed and the areas of the body that are exposed.

BOX 25-1 ▪ LIQUID EXPOSURE—NERVE AGENTS

Minimal exposure (droplet)

Local sweating
Muscle fasciculation
Nausea, vomiting, diarrhea
Generalized weakness: may persist for hours

Severe exposure

Briefly asymptomatic (1–30 min), then rapid, abrupt loss of consciousness
Convulsions
Generalized muscle fasciculation, flaccid paralysis
Copious secretions, bronchoconstriction, apnea
Death

BOX 25-2 ■ VAPOR EXPOSURE—NERVE AGENTS

Small exposure

Ocular (miosis, blurred vision, eye pain, conjunctival injection)
Nasal (rhinorrhea)
Pulmonary (bronchoconstriction, bronchorrhea, dyspnea)

Large exposure

Loss of consciousness after one breath
Convulsions
Severe bronchoconstriction with respiratory arrest, death

BOX 25-3 ■ OTHER CLINICAL SIGNS AND SYMPTOMS—NERVE AGENTS

Respiratory tract

Hypersalivation, weakness of tongue and pharyngeal muscles, paralysis
  of laryngeal muscles → stridor, respiratory muscle paralysis, direct
  depression of central respiratory drive (primary respiratory arrest)

Cardiovascular

Dependent on balance between nicotinic effects at autonomic ganglia and
  muscarinic effects at parasympathetic fibers → sinus tachydysrhythmias/
  hypertension (sympathetic tone predomination) or bradydysrhythmias/
  hypotension (parasympathetic)

CNS

Rapidly decreasing loss of consciousness, generalized seizures, headache,
  vertigo, paresthesias, insomnia, depression, emotional lability

---

Remember, **there may be an initial lack of signs and symptoms.**

- Liquid
  - Skin damage
  - Initial erythema with pruritis and burning followed by
    blistering (partial-thickness burn). With higher concen-
    trations, deep bullae or ulcers form, resembling scalded
    skin syndrome or toxic epidermal necrolysis. Blister fluid
    is nontoxic.
- Vapor
  - Upper respiratory tract (rarely lower respiratory or lung
    parenchyma)

- Damage within minutes, symptoms delayed 4–6 hr (up to 24 hr)
- Hemorrhagic inflammation and airway erosion
- Sinus congestion, sinusitis, sore throat, hoarseness, cough, dyspnea, respiratory distress, small and large airway obstruction secondary to epithelial sloughing and pseudomembrane formation
- Respiratory compromise up to several days after exposure if extensive mucosal involvement
- Other
  - Eye
- 4–8 hr postexposure: burning pain, foreign body sensation, photophobia, tearing, visual blurring, edema, conjunctivitis, ulceration
- GI
  - Abdominal pain, nausea, vomiting, diarrhea, weight loss
- Heme
  - Bone marrow suppression (begins 3–5 days postexposure), leukopenic nadir in 3–14 days

Choking Agents

- Phosgene
  - Delayed effects, possibly life-threatening if untreated
  - Eye and respiratory system irritation → dyspnea, pulmonary edema
  - Hypotension, hypovolemia
  - Bronchospasm, bronchorrhea
  - Right ventricular failure
  - Infection
  - Liquid phosgene can cause frostbite.
- Chlorine
  - See Box 25-4.
  - Respiratory symptoms may be immediate or delayed up to several hours after exposure.
  - Symptoms generally resolve within 6 hr after mild exposure but may continue for more than 24 hr after severe exposure.
  - Deterioration may continue for several hours.

Cyanides

- Immediately life-threatening
- Inhaled: convulsions, death
- Ingested: dizziness, nausea, vomiting, weakness, respiratory distress, loss of consciousness, convulsions, apnea, death

---

BOX 25-4 ▪ CHLORINE EXPOSURE

Pulmonary

Coughing, burning sensation in the chest, bloody sputum, pneumonitis, chest pain, dyspnea, respiratory distress, rales, bronchospasm and acute lung injury, respiratory arrest

Eye

Lacrimation, conjunctivitis, burning of the eyes, blepharospasm

Nose and throat

Burning in the nose and throat, sneezing, bloody nose, rhinorrhea, choking (cramps in the pharyngeal muscles)

Cardiovascular

Tachycardia, chest pain

Gastrointestinal

Nausea, vomiting, epigastric pain

Neurologic

Headache, dizziness, syncope

Psychiatric

Feeling of suffocation, anxiety

Other

Diaphoresis, muscle weakness, dermatitis

- Odor of bitter almonds: Less than 60% of the population can smell this odor.

Laboratory Evaluation

Nerve Agents

- Determine plasma and red blood cell cholinesterase **activities** (not levels).
    - There is poor correlation between cholinesterase values and clinical effects.
    - Pre-exposure cholinesterase activity would be helpful for diagnosis but typically is not available in emergency situations.

- Depression in excess of 50% activity is generally associated with severe symptoms.
- Remember, lab results are not necessary to initiate treatment.
- Obtain an ECG and institute continuous cardiac monitoring.
- Chest radiograph
- Monitor pulse oximetry and/or ABGs in all symptomatic patients.

Vesicating and Blistering Agents

Electrolytes, ABGs with respiratory involvement

Choking Agents

- Chest radiograph
- ABGs

Cyanides

See Chapter 15.

Treatment

- Personal protective equipment (PPE)
- Away from the hot zone, the primary concern is liquid contamination. If exposure was vapor only, there is little risk to hospital staff.
  - Level B or C PPE required; latex gloves and surgical masks are useless or inadequate.
- Decontamination: Should be done outside the emergency department.
  - Remove residual chemicals (including clothes and jewelry).
  - Irrigate with water, rinse with 0.5% hypochlorite solution (1 part hypochlorite [household bleach] to 9 parts water).
    - Avoid hot water and vigorous scrubbing.
- Supportive care: ABCs
- Specific antidotes if indicated (cyanide and nerve agent exposures), based on clinical criteria. No lab tests are available for rapid confirmation.

Nerve Agents

- Treatment is clinically based. Provide oxygen.
- See Table 25-2.
- 2-PAM should be given as soon as possible (concurrently with atropine); it is ineffective once phosphorylated AChE has aged. Rate of aging varies among agents.
    - Repeat 2-PAM hourly if toxicity persists or worsens. Toxicity rarely lasts more than 2 hr with adequate decontamination and appropriate initial therapy.
- Avoid succinylcholine because nerve agents prolong its paralytic effect.
- Termination of seizure activity may be secondary to flaccid paralysis from nerve agent and not because of "adequate" anticonvulsive treatment. A bedside EEG is needed to evaluate ongoing seizure activity.

Table 25-2 MANAGEMENT OF NERVE AGENT EXPOSURE

Treatment	Dose	Comment
Oxygen	Maintain satO$_2$ at 96% –100%	Via mask or ETT
Atropine	2 mg IV/IM/ET q 2–5 min	Mild to moderate symptoms
	5 mg IV/IM/ET Children: 0.02–0.05 mg/kg (0.1 mg minimum) IV/IM/ET	Severe symptoms. Titrate to clinical effect of dry secretions and elimination of bronchoconstriction.*
Pralidoxime chloride (2-PAM)	1–2 g IV (adult)	Administer slowly. Watch for hypertension during administration.
	Children: 15–25 mg/kg IV	May be given 1 mg IM (in 3 mL NS) if no IV access
Phentolamine	5 mg IV (adults), 1 mg IV (children)	
Benzodiazepines	Diazepam: 5–30 mg IV Children: 0.3–0.5 mg/kg Lorazepam: 2–10 mg IV (adults) Children: 0.05–0.1 mg/kg IV	Titrate to effect (consider prophylactic administration of diazepam).
Hemodialysis and hemoperfusion		If unresponsive to pharmacotherapy

Heart rate and pupil size are poor indicators of adequate atropinization. Up to 20 mg atropine may be required for the first day.

Vesicating and Blistering Agents

- Use level A PPE. This level is used when the greatest level of skin, respiratory, and eye protection is required (Box 25-5).
- Decontamination within 2 min of exposure: Remove clothing; wash skin with soap and water (0.5% hypochlorite solution or alkaline soap and water); for ocular exposure, irrigate eyes with saline/water.
- Supportive: ABCs; consider intubation for severe exposure because effects are delayed and persons with initial complaints still have additional injury.
- Moist air, mucolytics, *N*-acetylcysteine inhaled if respiratory complaints
- Narcotic analgesia
- Avoid overhydration (not the same fluid requirements as thermal burns).
- Adequate burn care
- Tetanus
- Ophthalmologic consultation for ocular burns

Choking Agents

- Supportive care/symptomatic treatment; monitor for nephrotoxicity.
- Close observation for at least 4 hr.

Cyanides

- Cyanide antidote kit

Box 25-5 ▪ Level A Equipment

1. Positive pressure, full face piece, self-contained breathing apparatus (SCBA) or positive pressure supplied air respirator with escape SCBA, approved by the National Institute for Occupational Safety and Health (NIOSH)
2. Totally-encapsulating chemical-protective suit
3. Coveralls (as needed)
4. Long underwear (as needed)
5. Gloves, outer, chemical-resistant
6. Gloves, inner, chemical-resistant
7. Boots, chemical-resistant, steel toe and shank
8. Hard hat (under suit) (as needed)
9. Disposable protective suit, gloves and boots (depending on suit construction, may be worn over totally-encapsulating suit)

- Amyl nitrite ampule inhaled for 30 sec/min until sodium nitrite can be given IV.
- Sodium nitrite 10 mL IV over 3 to 5 min (children: 0.15–0.33 mL/kg)
  - Goal is to increase methemoglobin, but not above 30%.
- Sodium thiosulfate 50 mL IV of 25% solution (children 1.65 mL/kg)

Special Considerations

- Mass casualty
  - Become familiar with your hospital's plan for handling chemical agents of terrorism and especially your role in the plan.
- Pregnancy
  - Pregnant patients with significant cyanide exposure can be treated the same as nonpregnant patients.

Admission Criteria

Nerve Agents

- Toxic effects peak within minutes to hours and resolve within 1 day.
- Asymptomatic with liquid exposure: Observe for 18 hr minimum.
- Symptomatic with liquid exposure: Admit and monitor for 1 day minimum.
- Vapor exposure: Peak effects occur prior to arrival at hospital. If only eye findings are present, patient may be discharged.

Mustards (Sulfur Mustard, Nitrogen Mustard)

- Admit to ICU and aggressive pulmonary care if patient has significant respiratory involvement.
- Admit to burn unit if significant dermal burns.
- Asymptomatic: Observe for 12 hr prior to discharge.

Choking Agents

Admit to ICU and aggressive pulmonary care if patient has significant respiratory involvement.

Cyanides

See Chapter 15.

Pearls and Pitfalls

- Be aware!
- Check your hospital pharmacy and Alert Plan for managing chemical warfare agents.
- Cyanide kills quickly if the dose is large enough. Those exposed to high concentrations will not make it to the ED.
- Check your cyanide antidote kit for expired drugs.
- In symptomatic nerve agent exposure, large doses of atropine may be needed.
- Start 2-PAM early in nerve agent exposures.

References and Suggested Readings

1. Ciottone G, Arnold J: CBRNE–Chemical Warfare Agents. www.emedicine.com, May 16, 2006.
2. Ellenhorn M, Schonwald S, Ordog G, et al, eds: *Ellenhorn's medical toxicology: diagnosis and treatment of human poisoning,* ed 2, Baltimore, 1997, Williams & Wilkins, pp 1270-1297.
3. Suchard JR: Chemical and biologic weapons. In Goldfrank L, Flomenbaum N, Lewin N, et al, eds: *Goldfrank's toxicologic emergencies,* ed 7, New York, 2002, McGraw-Hill, pp 1440-1441.

Toxicology
MNEMONICS AND
Useful PEARLS

Appendix A

Toxicology Mnemonics, Acronyms, and Pearls

Richard P. Lamon

This section includes tidbits and "mind-tingling" quips and pearls that the authors have heard throughout our careers from mentors and attending physicians. The exact origins or sources have been misplaced or are unknown.

These are helpful tools to use in daily practice. Remember, these mnemonics are not all encompassing; there may be other toxins to include. Play with this list and add new toxins when you encounter them, keeping the basic mnemonic whenever possible.

Mnemonics and Acronyms

1. Alteration of consciousness: "Do the **DONT**"

    D   Dextrose

    O   Oxygen

    N   Narcan

    T   Thiamine

(It's been suggested that you don't automatically "Do the DON'T," but think about doing it when you see someone with altered consciousness.)

2. Substances causing seizures: **"WITH LA COPS"**

   W   Withdrawal *(alcohol, benzodiazepine, GHB, opiates in neonates only)*

   I   Isoniazid, iron, insulin, industrial acids, and inhalants

   T   Theophylline, tricyclics, tramadol

   H   Hypoglycemics, Haldol, hemlock, hydrazines

   L   Lead, lithium, local anesthetics, lindane

   A   Anticholinergics, anticonvulsants, antibiotics (quinolones, imipenem, dapsone)

   C   Carbon monoxide, cocaine, cyanide, cholinergics, camphor

   O   Organophosphates

   P   Phencyclidine (PCP), propoxyphene, propranolol, phenylpropanolamine

   S   Strychnine, salicylates, sympathomimetics, SSRI (fluoxetine, citalopram)

NOTE: There are many other mnemonics relating to substances causing seizures:

- **OTIS CAMPBELL** (if you're old enough to have watched "The Andy Griffith Show," this might mean something)
- **WITHDRAWALS**
- **PLASTIC (4)** (the "4" is for the 4 agents beginning with each letter).

3. Substances causing nystagmus: **"SALEM TIP"**

   S   Sedative hypnotics, solvents

   A   Alcohols

   L   Lithium

   E   Ethylene glycol, ethanol

   M   Methanol

   T   Thiamine depletion, Tegretol

   I   Isopropanol

   P   PCP, phenytoin

4. Radiopaque substances: **"BET A CHIP"**

   B   Barium

   E   Enteric-coated tablets

   T   Tricyclics

   A   Antihistamines

   C   Condoms, chloral hydrate, calcium

   H   Heavy metals

- I   Iodine
- P   Potassium, phenothiazines

5. Substances forming concretions: **"BIG-O-MESS"**
   - B   Barbiturates
   - I   Iron
   - G   Glutethimide
   - O   Opiates
   - M   Meprobamate
   - E   Extended-release tablets
   - S   Sustained-release preparations
   - S   Salicylates

NOTE: In some areas, concretions are known as "pharmaco-bezoars." There has been recent controversy as to whether non-enteric coated aspirin really cause concretion.

6. Dangerous additives to hydrocarbons: **"CHAMP"**
   - C   Camphor
   - H   Halogenated hydrocarbons
   - A   Aromatics
   - M   Metals
   - P   Pesticides

7. Cholinergic toxidrome (anticholinesterase inhibitors): **"SLUG BAM"**
   - S   Salivation, secretions, sweating
   - L   Lacrimation
   - U   Urination
   - G   Gastrointestinal upset
   - B   Bradycardia, bronchoconstriction
   - A   Abdominal cramps
   - M   Miosis

   Cholinergic toxidrome: **"SLUDGE"**
   - S   Salivation
   - L   Lacrimation
   - U   Urination
   - D   Diarrhea, diaphoresis
   - G   Gastrointestinal upset
   - E   Emesis

Cholinergic toxidrome: **"DUMBELS"**

D   Defecation

U   Urination

M   Miosis

B   Bronchorrhea, bradycardia

E   Emesis

L   Lacrimation

S   Salivation, sweating

8. Nicotinic effects of anticholinesterase inhibitors: **"M-T-W-tH-F"**

M   Mydriasis, muscle twitching

T   Tachycardia

W   Weakness

tH   Hypertension, hyperglycemia

F   Fasciculations

9. Causes of increased anion gap metabolic acidosis: **"A MUD PILE CAT"**

A   ASA

M   Methanol

U   Uremia

D   DKA

P   Paraldehyde, phenformin

I   INH, iron, ibuprofen, inhalant abuse

L   Lactic acidosis

E   Ethylene glycol

C   Carbon monoxide, cyanide, caffeine, cocaine

A   Acetaminophen (>600 µg/ml), alcohol ketoacidosis

T   Theophylline, toluene

Others: benzyl alcohol, metaldehyde, formaldehyde, H_2S

You should know how to calculate the anion gap. Don't rely on the lab!

$$\text{Anion gap} = Na - (Cl + HCO_3)$$

(In most labs, the normal is within the range of 8 to 12.)

This list is somewhat more complete than your usual MUDPILES, isn't it?

NOTE: Substances and conditions causing a **decreased** anion gap: bromide, lithium, hypermagnesemia, hypercalcemia, and diabetes.

10. Substances causing an osmolal gap: **"MAD GAS"**

    M   Mannitol

    A   Alcohols (methanol, ethylene glycol, isopropanol, ethanol)

    D   DMSO (dimethylsulfoxide), dyes, diuretics

    G   Glycerol

    A   Acetone

    S   Sorbitol

    Substances causing an osmolal gap: **"ME DIES"**

    M   Methanol

    E   Ethylene glycol

    D   DMSO, dyes, diuretics

    I   Isopropyl and metabolites (acetone)

    E   Ethanol

    S   Sugars

Serum osmolality is normally 285-295 mOsm/L. The difference between the measured and the calculated osmolality is the osmolal gap. The measured osmolality should not exceed the predicted by more than 10 mOsm/L. A difference of more than 10 mOsm/L is considered an osmolal gap. The formula for calculating the osmolality is

$$\text{Calculated Osmolality} = 2 \times Na + glucose/18 + BUN/2.8$$

11. Causes of prolongation of QT: **"PF TORSADES"**

    P   Phosphides, Propulsid, pentamidine, pimozide

    F   Fluorides, fluoxetine

    T   TCA, thioridazine

    O   Organic mercury, opioids (heroin), octreotide

    R   Rhythm-controllers (Class Ia, III antidysrhythmics)

    S   Scorpion/spider venom

    A   Arsenic, antihistamines (Hismanal, Seldane), antimalarial

    D   Darvocet

    E   Emetic (ipecac), electrolytes (MG, K, Ca—low)

    S   Severe hypothermia and bradycardia

    Others: Lithium, Celexa, Effexor (with QRS increase), sertraline

12. Drugs and conditions causing pinpoint pupils: **"COPS"**

    C   Clonidine

    O   Organophosphate, olanzapine, opiates

    P   Pilocarpine, pontine hemorrhage

    S   Sedatives

13. Substances causing garlic odor on breath: **"TOADS P"**

    T Thallium

    O Organophosphates

    A Arsenic

    D DMSO

    S Selenium

    P Phosphorous

Think: TOAD'S Pee smells like garlic!

14. Salicylate toxidrome: **"ASPIRIN"**

    A Altered mental status (lethargy to coma)

    S Sweating

    P Pulmonary edema

    I Irritability

    R Ringing in ears

    I Increased respirations, temperature, heart rate

    N Nausea and vomiting

Toxin-Induced Changes in Vital Signs

1. Toxins causing *bradycardia:* **"PACED"**

   P Propranolol or other beta blockers, poppies (opiates)

   A Anticholinesterase drugs

   C Clonidine, calcium channel blockers, ciguatera poisoning

   E Ethanol or other alcohols, ergotamine

   D Digoxin

   Other: GHB

2. Toxins causing *tachycardia:* **"FAST"**

   F Free base or other forms of cocaine

   A Anticholinergics

   S Sympathomimetics (ephedrine, amphetamines), solvent abuse

   T Theophylline, thyroid hormone

3. Toxins causing *hypothermia:* **"COOLS"**

   C Carbon monoxide, clonidine

   O Opiates

   O Oral hypoglycemics, insulin

   L Liquor

   S Sedative-hypnotics

4. Toxins and conditions causing *hyperthermia:* **"NASA"**

   N   Nicotine, neuroleptic malignant syndrome

   A   Antihistamines

   S   Salicylates, sympathomimetics, serotonin syndrome

   A   Anticholinergics, antidepressants

5. Toxins causing *hypotension:* **"CRASH"**

   C   Clonidine, calcium channel blockers (and beta blockers)

   R   Reserpine or other antihypertensives

   A   Antidepressants, aminophylline, alcohol

   S   Sedative-hypnotics

   H   Heroin and other opiates

6. Toxins causing *hypertension:* **"CT SCAN"**

   C   Cocaine

   T   Thyroid supplements

   S   Sympathomimetics

   C   Caffeine

   A   Anticholinergics, amphetamines

   N   Nicotine

7. Toxins causing *increased respiratory rate:* **"PANT"**

   P   PCP, paraquat, pneumonitis (chemical)

   A   ASA and other salicylates, amphetamines

   N   Noncardiogenic pulmonary edema

   T   Toxin-induced metabolic acidosis

8. Toxins causing *decreased respiratory rate:* **"SLOW"**

   S   Sedative hypnotic, strychnine, snakes

   L   Liquor

   O   Opiates, organophosphates

   W   Weed (marijuana)

   Others: nicotine, clonidine, chlorinated hydrocarbons

9. Toxins causing *diaphoretic skin:* **"SOAP"**

   S   Sympathomimetics

   O   Organophosphates

   A   ASA or other salicylates

   P   Phencyclidine (PCP)

10. Toxins causing *dry skin:* **"AA"** (like Alcoholics Anonymous)

   A   Antihistamines

   A   Anticholinergics

Lists

1. Toxins causing coma
   Alcohols
   Anticholinergics
   Arsenic
   Beta blockers
   Carbon monoxide
   Cholinergic agents
   Cyclic antidepressants
   Lead, lithium
   Opioids
   PCP
   Phenothiazines
   Salicylates
   Sedative hypnotics

2. Toxins causing changes in the pupils
   Miosis:
   Cholinergics
   Clonidine
   Nicotine
   Opioids (except meperidine [Demerol])
   PCP
   Phenothiazines
   Mydriasis:
   Anticholinergics
   Glutethimide
   Meperidine
   Sympathomimetics
   Withdrawal

3. Toxins causing changes in respirations
   Decreased respirations:
   Alcohols
   Barbiturates
   Benzodiazepine
   Opioids

Increased respirations:

CO

CN

Drug-induced hepatic failure

Drug-induced metabolic acidosis

Drug-induced methemoglobinemia

Salicylates

4. Toxins causing changes in heart rate

Tachycardia:

Anticholinergics

Antihistamines

Cyclic antidepressants

PCP

Quetiapine

Sympathomimetics: cocaine, amphetamine, clonidine, Theophylline, withdrawal states

Bradycardia:

Alpha blockers

Beta blockers

Calcium channel blockers

Cardiac glycosides

Cholinergics

Cyanide

Nicotine

Parasympathomimetics

5. Toxins causing changes in blood pressure

Hypertension: Similar to those causing tachycardia

Anticholinergics

MAO inhibitors

Phencyclidine

Sympathomimetics

Withdrawal

Hypotension:

CO

CN

Cyclic antidepressants

Iron

Nitrites (nitrates)

Opioids

Phenothiazines

Sedative-hypnotics

Theophylline

6. Toxins causing changes in temperature

Hyperthermia:

Anticholinergics

Dinitrophenols

MAOIs

Metals

Neuroleptics

PCP

Phenothiazines

Salicylates

Sympathomimetics

Withdrawal states

Hypothermia:

Beta blockers

Cholinergics

CO

Ethanol

Hypoglycemics

Sedative-hypnotics

7. Toxins causing odor of breath

Acetone:

Ethanol

Isopropanol

Ketosis

Salicylates

Almonds:

Amygdalin

Apricot pits

Cyanide

Laetrile

Garlic:

Arsenic

Arsine gas

DMSO

Organophosphates

Phosphorous

Thallium

Peanuts:

Rodenticides

Vacor

Pears:

Chloral hydrate

Paraldehyde

Rotten eggs:

Hydrogen sulfide

Mercaptans

Sewer gas

Wintergreen:

Salicylates (oil of wintergreen)

Toxins Affecting the Skin

1. Toxins causing **bullous lesions** of the skin

   Benzodiazepines

   Blistering agents

   Carbon monoxide

   Caustic agents

   Hydrocarbons

   Sedative hypnotics

   Snake bite

   Spider bite

   Tricyclic antidepressants

2. Toxins requiring skin **decontamination**

   Aniline dyes

   Caustics

   Cyanide

   DMSO

Hydrocarbons

Mace

Methanol

Pesticides

Radiation

3. Toxins causing **damp** skin

Aspirin and other salicylates

Organophosphates

Phencyclidine (PCP)

Sympathomimetics

4. Toxins causing **dry** skin

Antihistamines

Anticholinergics

5. Toxins causing **flushed** skin

Anticholinergics

Boric acid

CN (rare)

CO (r are)

6. Toxins causing **cyanosis**

Aniline dyes

Dapsone

Ergotamine

Lidocaine, benzocaine

Nitrates

Nitrites

Phenazopyridine

Other: any agent causing hypoxia, hypotension, methemoglo-binemia

Toxidromes

Stimulant toxidrome:

Restlessness

Excessive speech

Excessive motor activity

Tremor

Insomnia

Tachycardia

Hallucinations

Sedative-hypnotic toxidrome:

Sedation

Confusion

Delirium

Hallucinations

Coma

Paresthesias

Dysesthesias

Diplopia

Blurred vision

Slurred speech

Ataxia

Nystagmus

Opiate toxidrome:

Altered mental status

Miosis

Unresponsiveness

Shallow respirations

Slow respiratory rate

Bradycardia

Decreased bowel sounds

Hypothermia

Anticholinergic toxidrome:

Fever

Ileus

Flushing

Tachycardia

Urinary retention

Dry skin

Blurred vision

Mydriasis

Decreased bowel sounds

Myoclonus

Choreoathetosis

Psychosis

Hallucinations

Seizures

Coma (Hot as a hare, Dry as a bone, Red as a beet, Blind as a bat, Mad as a hatter)

Cholinergic toxidrome:

Salivation

Lacrimation

Urination

Defecation

Gastrointestinal distress (diarrhea)

Emesis

Bronchorrhea, bradycardia

Table 1 DRUG WITH ANTIDOTES	
Drug	**Antidote**
Acetaminophen	*N*-acetylcysteine
Anticholinergics	Physostigmine
Arsenic	BAL, penicillamine
Beta blockers	Glucagon
Bromides	Chlorides
Carbon monoxide	Oxygen
Coumadin	Vitamin K
Cyanide	Nitrite, thiosulfate (Lilly Kit)
Digoxin	Fab antibodies
Ethylene glycol	Ethyl alcohol and fomepizole
Iron	Deferoxamine
Isoniazid (INH)	Pyridoxine
Lead	BAL, Ca EDTA, penicillamine
Mercury	Penicillamine, BAL
Methanol	Ethanol and (?) fomepizole
Methemoglobinemia	Methylene blue
Opiates	Naloxone
Organophosphates	Atropine, PAM
Tricyclics	Alkalinization

BAL, British anti-lewisite ; EDTA, ethylenediaminetetraacetic acid; PAM, pralidoxime.

Appendix B

The Toxicology Lab

Kristin Engebretsen

When to Order Toxicology Screens

Many factors should be considered prior to ordering a toxicology screen. The following questions should be asked prior to obtaining any toxicology labs:

1. Do you want a qualitative or a quantitative screen?
2. Is there a predictable relationship between concentration and adverse effects?
3. What is the analytical time required to obtain the laboratory result?
4. Will the result influence your clinical practice?

You must first decide if a qualitative or quantitative result is required (i.e., do you just want to know if the drug is present [qualitative], or do you need to know the concentration of the drug present [quantitative]). Most drugs can be detected and qualitatively identified through a urine specimen.

However, if you are considering obtaining a quantitative result on the toxin, then serum is used for the majority of toxins. Prior to obtaining a serum concentration of the toxin, you should ask yourself the following question:

Can the level obtained be used to accurately predict toxicity in a patient?
- If not, there is really no reason to obtain the level.
- Predictable correlations between concentrations and toxicity are the exception in most cases, not the rule. This may be due to multiple reasons such as:

- The toxic effects are local, not systemic (e.g., caustics).
- Patients may develop tolerances to drugs, allowing some patients to tolerate very large amounts with minimal symptoms whereas other patients may exhibit toxicity even with small doses (e.g., cocaine).
- The pharmacokinetics or pharmacodynamics for therapeutic dosing may be different from overdose situations (e.g., theophylline, which changes from first order elimination at therapeutic doses to zero order in overdose).
- The reaction may be idiosyncratic or not dose dependent.
- The data may just not be available secondary to a lack of toxicology research.
- Of those toxins that have been well studied, fewer than two dozen actually have demonstrated reliable correlations between body fluids and toxicity effects.[1]
- The most commonly obtained serum concentrations include acetaminophen, salicylates, methanol, ethylene glycol, ethanol, anticonvulsants, iron, and lithium.

Techniques Used

Current methods of drug analysis include but are not limited to the following:

1. Chromatography: thin layer (TLC), Gas (GC), or high-performance liquid (HPLC)
2. Immunoassay: enzyme immunoassay (EIA or EMIT), fluorescence polarization, and immunoaggregation
3. Chemical: spot
4. Spectrometry: mass-spectrometry

Currently, most rapid toxicology screens use immunoassay techniques. However, if a drug is detected, it should always be confirmed by a second method with high specificity for that drug.

Time Factors

Once you determine that you need to obtain either a qualitative or quantitative level, then you must determine where you will send the sample for testing. Your own hospital or local laboratory may be able to do some of the testing; however, if they are not common assays or if you are practicing at a smaller hospital, your laboratory may not be able to test for the substances. Samples must then be sent to a toxicology lab. This often results in long turnaround times (usually days). Standard turnaround times if a sample is to be sent to another lab are frequently 3 days or longer. Therefore, the lab, although attainable, may be useless in the treatment of the patient because the critical time period of the toxin will have passed. If a level is required to determine treatment (e.g., acetaminophen or ethylene glycol levels) but cannot be obtained in the needed timeframe, the patient may need to be transferred to a larger hospital with more advanced laboratory capabilities, treatment may need to be initiated before the laboratory results have returned, or both. Finally, even in large hospitals with excellent laboratory capabilities, laboratory results may be delayed due to the "stat phenomena" (i.e., all labs are ordered stat, thus delaying those labs that truly should take priority).

Limitations: Blind Spots and False Negatives

Remember that there are both rapid urine toxicology screens and comprehensive urine toxicology screens. The rapid screens usually only detect five or six common substances. This screen may vary by hospital but frequently tests for agents such as cocaine, tricyclic antidepressants, opiates, PCP, benzodiazepines, and amphetamines.

- However, one must realize that not all benzodiazepines will be detected by this screen.
  - It is extremely important to consult your toxicology laboratory to determine what the assay will detect.
  - Newer agents such as clonazepam, lorazepam, and midazolam are frequently not detected by some assays.
  - Opiates also may cause much confusion because methadone and some synthetic opiates such as propoxyphene frequently may not be detected by certain assays.
  - Do not assume that all drugs of a class are covered; doing so may lead you to a "misdiagnosis."

For toxicology screening blind spots, see Boxes 1 and 2. For serum drug screens, see Boxes 3 and 4. For urine drug screens, see Boxes 5 and 6. For toxicology tests frequently performed by general chemistry labs, see Box 7.

Box 1 ▪ Drugs Frequently Undetected by Toxicology Screens

Antidepressants: Trazodone, paroxetine, fluoxetine, venlafaxine, bupropion
Antimanic: Lithium
Antipsychotics: Haloperidol, thiothixene, risperidone, olanzapine, clozapine, ziprasidone, quetiapine, amoxapine
MAO Inhibitors: Phenelzine
Opioids: Diphenoxylate, fentanyl, methadone
Sedative-hypnotics: Chloral hydrate, paraldehyde, newer benzodiazepines (Clonazepam, Versed, Rohypnol)
Others: GHB, INH, diuretics, antihistamines (Benadryl), anticholinergics, colchicine, antihypertensives, newer antiepileptics (Gabapentin), antiarrhythmics, ethylene glycol, ergots, plants, venoms, strychnine, SSRIs (selective serotonin reuptake inhibitors), methemoglobin, methanol, MDMA (ecstasy), anticoagulants, β-agonists, β-antagonists, calcium channel blockers, carbon monoxide, clonidine, cyanide, digoxin, gamma hydroxybutyrate, heavy metals, hypoglycemic agents, iron, isopropyl alcohol, ketamine

Box 2 ▪ Substances Frequently Undetected by Toxicology Screens

Biologic toxins: Mushrooms, plants, strychnine
Hallucinogens: LSD, mescaline
Metals: Lead, arsenic, mercury, iron
Pesticides: Cholinesterase inhibitors, halogenated hydrocarbons
Solvents: Benzene, trichloroethylene, 1-1-1-trichloroethane
Others: CO, CN, camphor, borate, fluoride, strychnine

Box 3 ▪ Serum Screens: Specific Drugs

Acetaminophen >50 μg/ml
Amitriptyline
Barbiturates
Caffeine
Carbamazepine
Carisoprodol
Chlordiazepoxide (Librium)
Chlorpheniramine
Chlorpromazine
Chlorzoxazone
Clomipramine (Tranxene)
Clorazepate
Cocaine

Cyclobenzaprine (Flexeril)
Diazepam
Doxepin
Ethchlorvynol
Ethosuximide
Flurazepam
Glutethimide
Ibuprofen
Imipramine
Maprotiline
Meprobamate
Methaqualone
Methyprylon

Pentazocine
Phenacetin
Phenylbutazone
Phenytoin
Primidone
Propoxyphene
Propranolol
Protriptyline
Salicylate*
Theophylline
Valproic acid

* Drug found on serum screen only.

Box 4 ▪ Serum Screens: Volatiles			
Acetone	Ethanol	Isopropanol	Methanol

▪ Laboratory Information

Pulmonary Labs

Pulmonary labs typically perform the following tests:
- COhgb
- Methgb

Send-Out Labs

The following is a list of laboratories that may be able to perform toxicologic analyses. Labs may differ on what they can and cannot analyze. It is best to contact the lab directly for services provided, special requirements in sending samples, and time required.

MedTox Scientific, Inc.

West County Rd. D

St. Paul, MN 55112

(T) 800-832-3244

Comments: SMHSA-certified drug testing laboratory; able to do pharmaceutical, drugs of abuse, and employment drug screening.

Pacific Toxicology Laboratories

6160 Variel Ave.

Woodland Hills, CA 91367

(T) 800-328-6942

info@pactox.com or clientservices@pactox.com

Comments: Serology, immunology, chemistry, hematology, and forensic toxicology testing; able to test for pesticides and drugs of abuse.

Product Safety Laboratories (PSL)

2394 Route 130

Dayton, NJ 08810

(T) 732-438-5100

BOX 5 ▪ URINE SCREENS: SPECIFIC DRUGS

Acetaminophen
Amitriptyline
Amobarbital
Amphetamine
  (Dextroamphetamine
  and methamphetamine)
Atenolol
Azacyclonol
Barbital
Butalbital
Caffeine
Carbamazepine (Tegretol)
Carisoprodol
Chlorpheniramine
Chlorpromazine
Chlorzoxazone
Clomipramine
Cocaine + methylester
  ecgonine
Codeine
Cotinine
Cyclobenzaprine
Desipramine
Diazepam
Diphenhydramine
Doxepin
Doxylamine

Ephedrine
Ethchlorvynol
Ethosuximide
Fluoxetine (Prozac)
Flurazepam
Glutethimide
Hydrocodone
Ibuprofen
Imipramine
Ketamine
Labetalol
Lidocaine
Loxapine
Maprotiline
Meperidine
Mephobarbital
Meprobamate
Methadone
Methapyrilene
Methaqualone
Methorphan
Methylphenidate
Methylprylon
Morphine
Nicotine
Nordiazepam
Nortriptyline

Oxycodone
Pentobarbital
Phenacetin
Pentazocine
Phencyclidine
Phendimetrazine
Phenmetrazine
Phenobarbital
Phentermine
Phenylpropanolamine
Phenytoin
Primidone (Mysoline)
Propranolol
Protriptyline
Pseudoephedrine
Pyrilamine
Secobarbital
THC metabolite
Theophylline
Thiopental
  (Pentothal)
Tranylcypromine
Trimipramine
Tripelennamine
Triprolidine
Valproic acid

Italicized drugs *are those that are also found on serum screen.*

BOX 6 ▪ URINE SCREEN: NONSPECIFIC CLASS BY EMIT

Amphetamines	Benzodiazepines	Opioids	THC metabolite
Barbiturates	Cocaine metabolites	PCP	

BOX 7 ▪ TOXICOLOGY TESTS DONE BY GENERAL CHEMISTRY LAB

Acetaminophen	Lactate	Phenytoin
Aminoglycosides	Lidocaine	Quinidine
Carbamazepine	Lithium	Salicylate
Digoxin	NAPA and procainamide	Theophylline
Iron	Phenobarbital	Valproic acid

(F) 732-355-3275

psl@productsafetylabs.com

Comments: Pharmacologic, pesticide, and toxicologic testing.

Rocky Mountain Instrumental Laboratories, Inc.

108 Coronado Ct.

Ft. Collins, CO 80525

(T) 970-266-8108

rklantz@rockylab.com

Comments: Offers testing for both common and uncommon pharmaceuticals in both dosage forms and biosamples. Does not offer STAT services but is quite willing to develop assays for uncommon compounds or at very low levels. Inspected by the FDA, CLIA, and the Colorado Department of Health.

Reference

1. Rainey PM: Laboratory principles and techniques for evaluation of the poisoned or overdosed patient. In Goldfrank LR, Flomenbaum NE, Lewin NA, et al, eds: *Goldfrank's toxicological emergencies*, ed 7, New York, 2002, McGraw-Hill, pp 69-93.

A p p e n d i x C

Antidotes

James Wood

An antidote is an agent used to neutralize or counteract the effects of a poison. Table 2 presents a list of antidotes.

Pearls and Pitfalls

- Monitor for pulmonary edema and acute withdrawal syndrome when using Narcan.
- Methylene blue functions as a pro-oxidant compound if it is used at too high a dose and can actually cause methemoglobinemia.
- Treat cyanide poisonings with sodium thiosulfate alone if the patient was also exposed to carbon monoxide. Nitrites can cause methemoglobinemia.
- When treating cholinergic toxicity, administer atropine until patient develops anticholinergic symptoms (e.g., fever, flushing, redness, drying).

Table 2 ANTIDOTES

Antidote	Ingestion	Notes
N-acetylcysteine	Acetaminophen	Load with 140 mg/kg, then 70 mg kg q 4 hr PO × 17 doses; should be administered within 8 hr of ingestion for peak effect; repeat dose if emesis within 1 hr of administration; IV NAC *may* be preferable in pregnant patients (see Chapter 2, "Acetaminophen"). Refer to Rumack nomogram for indications.
Atropine	Organophosphates	2–4 mg IV q 5–10 min prn (adult), 0.05 mg/kg IV q 5 min prn (children); treat until anticholinergic symptoms noted (i.e., drying).
Benztropine	Phenothiazines	2 mg IM/IV in adults; 0.02 mg/kg, 1 mg maximum in children >3 yrs for dystonic reactions.
Calcium	Beta blocker, calcium channel blocker	1 g calcium chloride or 3 g calcium gluconate IV, repeat q 10–20 min for 3–4 doses, monitor serum calcium for repeat doses; caution in patients taking digoxin.
Calcium disodium edetate (EDTA)	Lead	1000–1500 mg/M²/day IV continuous infusion or divided and given over 1 hr every 6 hr; administer BAL first for high levels or encephalopathy; maintain adequate urine output to protect against nephrotoxicity.
Calcium gluconate	Hydrofluoric acid	Topical, subcutaneous, or intra-arterial administration for burns.
Cyanide antidote kit	Cyanide	Give amyl nitrite pearls while obtaining IV access, then sodium nitrite IV (10 mL adults, 0.33 mL/kg children), sodium thiosulfate IV (50 mL adult, 1.65 mL/kg children).

Continued

Table 2 ANTIDOTES—CONT'D		
Antidote	Ingestion	Notes
Deferoxamine	Iron	15 mg/kg/hr IV up to 24 hours; pulmonary, ocular, and ototoxicity described for longer administrations; consider whole bowel irrigation.
Digoxin Fab fragments	Digoxin, digitoxin, oleander, foxglove	Known digoxin level: # vials = (digoxin serum level × patient weight)/100. Unknown level: 10–20 vials IV; serum dig. levels not useful after Digibind administration, follow clinical response.
Dimercaprol (BAL)	Arsenic, mercury, lead	3 mg/kg deep IM q 4–6 hr for 2 days, then q 12 hr for 7–10 days; avoid in patients with peanut allergies; alkalinization of urine may protect kidneys during therapy.
Diphenhydramine	Phenothiazines	25–50 mg PO/IM/IV q 4–6 hr for akathisia and dystonic reaction.
DMSA	Lead (arsenic, mercury—not FDA approved)	10 mg/kg PO tid × 5 days in adults; 1050 mg/m^2/day PO × 5 days in children; more selective and less toxic than EDTA or BAL; can be given concomitantly with iron.
Ethanol	Ethylene glycol, methanol	Load with 800 mg/kg, then 1–1.5 mg/kg/hr; maintain blood alcohol level at 100–150 mg/dL; hypertonic solution, therefore monitor for possible hyponatremia.
Flumazenil	Benzodiazepines	0.2 mg IV given over 30 sec; if no response, 0.3 mg over 30 sec, if still no response, then 0.5 mg IV q 1 min to maximum 3-mg dose. Avoid in patients with known seizure disorder, ingestion of potential seizure-provoking agent (heterocyclic antidepressants), chronic benzodiazepine use, head trauma.

Fomepizole (4-MP)	Ethylene glycol, methanol	Load 15 mg/kg, then 10 mg/kg q 12 hr × 4 doses, then increase to 15 mg/kg q 12 hr PRN.
Glucagon	Beta blockers, calcium channel blockers	Initial IV bolus of 50 µg/kg over 1 min followed by continuous infusion of 2–5 mg/hr tapering as patient improves. Higher doses may be required (up to 10 mg in an adult) if initial dose is inadequate; dose-dependent nausea and vomiting.
Hyperbaric oxygen	CO poisoning	Controversial; consider use for patients with severe exposure, neurologic deficits, or pregnant women and children.
Methylene blue	Nitrites	1–2 mg/kg IV in adults, 0.3–1 mg/kg in children administered over 5 min; ineffective in patients with G-6-PD deficiency; consider exchange transfusion or hyperbaric oxygen therapy.
Naloxone	Opioids	0.4 –2 mg IV, monitor for return of respiratory depression, may need to give additional bolus or continuous infusion for long-acting opioids; may also be given IM or SQ.
Physostigmine	Atropine	1–2 mg IV given over 5 min in adults, 0.02 mg/kg in children; avoid rapid administration, which may cause bradycardia, hypersalivation, or seizures; should not be used in TCA overdose.
Pralidoxime (2-PAM)	Organophosphates	1–2 g IV over 30 min for adults, 20–40 mg/kg for children; only currently available cholinesterase-reactivating agent in U.S.; must be given within 48 hr of exposure; should always be used in conjunction with atropine.

Continued

Table 2 ANTIDOTES—CONT'D		
Antidote	Ingestion	Notes
Protamine	Heparin	25–50 mg IV; risk of hypotension, anaphylactic reaction; excess protamine can have anticoagulant effect.
Prussian blue (aka ferric ferrocyanide)	Thallium	Acts as an ion-exchange resin: thallium is exchanged for potassium in the gastrointestinal lumen, producing a nonabsorbable complex. The complex is then excreted in the feces. The recommended dose is 250 mg/kg/24 hr in 4 divided doses PO or NG. (Some authors maintain that activated charcoal is as effective.)
Pyridoxine	Isoniazid	Administer g/g INH ingestion (max. 5 g).
Sodium bicarbonate	Phenobarbital, chlorpropamide, salicylates, heterocyclic antidepressants	1–2 mEq/kg IV bolus, then continuous infusion of 100 mEq in 1 L D5W to maintain urine pH >7.45.
Vitamin K$_1$	Coumadin	Optimal dose not established. Administer 2.5–10 mg orally or by slow (1 mg/min) IV. Oral route preferred due to risk of anaphylactoid reaction with IV administration. Manage significant bleeding acutely with FFP.

NAC, *N-acetylcysteine;* BAL, *British anti-Lewisite;* TCA, *tricyclic antidepressant;* INH, *isoniazid;* FFP, *fresh frozen plasma.*

Appendix D

Street Names for Drugs of Abuse

Carson R. Harris

Having a little knowledge of street terminology may help you understand some of the "drug-speak" you may encounter during the evaluation of the drug abuse patient. Street names for drugs and drug paraphernalia are always changing. Certain terms may be used more often depending on location. When in doubt, multiple Internet sources provide street names for abused drugs.

Drug Abuse Terminology 101

Table 3 Street Names for Drugs of Abuse

Street Names	Abused Drug/Interpretation
A	LSD; amphetamine
Acapulco gold	Marijuana from southwestern Mexico
Acapulco red	Marijuana
Ace	Marijuana; PCP
Acid	LSD
AD	PCP
Adam	MDMA
African black	Marijuana
African bush	Marijuana
African woodbine	Marijuana cigarette
Ah-pen-yen	Opium
Aimies	Amphetamine; amyl nitrite
AIP	Heroin from Afghanistan, Iran, Pakistan

Table 3 STREET NAMES FOR DRUGS OF ABUSE—CONT'D	
Street Names	**Abused Drug/Interpretation**
Airplane	Marijuana
Alice B. Toklas	Marijuana brownie
Ames	Amyl nitrite
Amidone	Methadone
Amoeba	PCP
Amp	Amphetamine
Amp joint	Marijuana cigarette laced with some form of narcotic or formaldehyde
AMT	Dimethyltryptamine
Amys	Amyl nitrate
Anadrol	Oral steroid
Anatrofin	Injectable steroid
Anavar	Oral steroid
Angel	PCP
Angel dust, hair, mist, poke	PCP
Angie	Cocaine
Angola	Marijuana
Animal	LSD
Animal trank	PCP
Animal tranquilizer	PCP
Antifreeze	Heroin
Apache	Fentanyl
Apple jacks	Crack
Aries	Heroin
Aroma of men	Isobutyl nitrite
Ashes	Marijuana
Atom bomb	Marijuana and heroin
Atshitshi	Marijuana
Aunt Hazel	Heroin
Aunt Mary	Marijuana
Aunt Nora	Cocaine
Auntie	Opium
Auntie Emma	Opium
Aurora borealis	PCP
B.J.s	Crack
B40	Cigar laced with marijuana and dipped in malt liquor
Baby	Marijuana
Baby bhang	Marijuana
Baby T	Crack
Backbreakers	LSD and strychnine
Backjack	To inject opium
Backwards	Depressant

Bad	Crack
Bad bundle	Inferior-quality heroin
Bad seed	Peyote; heroin; marijuana
Bagging	Inhalant abuse by inhaling the fumes from a plastic bag
Bale	Marijuana
Ball	Crack
Ballot	Heroin
Bam	Depressant; amphetamine
Bambalacha	Marijuana
Bambs	Depressant
Bang	To inject a drug; inhalant
Bank bandit pills	Depressant
Bar	Marijuana
Barb	Depressant
Barbies	Depressant
Barbs	Cocaine
Barrels	LSD
Base	Cocaine; crack, freebasing
Baseball	Crack
Bash	Marijuana
Basuco	Cocaine; coca paste residue sprinkled on marijuana or regular cigarette
Bathtub speed	Methcathinone
Battery acid	LSD
Batu	Smokeable methamphetamine
Bazooka	Cocaine; crack
Bazulco	Cocaine sulfate
Beam me up Scottie	Crack dipped in PCP
Beans	Amphetamine; depressant; mescaline
Beast	LSD
Beast, the	Heroin
Beautiful boulders	Crack
Beavis and Butthead	LSD blotter acid
Bebe	Crack
Beemers	Crack
Beiging	Chemicals altering cocaine to make it appear a higher purity
Belladonna	PCP
Belushi	Cocaine and heroin
Belyando spruce	Marijuana
Bennie	Amphetamine
Benz	Amphetamine
Bernice	Cocaine
Bernie	Cocaine
Bernie's flakes	Cocaine

Continued

Table 3 STREET NAMES FOR DRUGS OF ABUSE—CONT'D

Street Names	Abused Drug/Interpretation
Bernie's gold dust	Cocaine
Bhang	Marijuana, Indian term
Big 8	$\frac{1}{8}$ kilogram of crack
Big bag	Heroin
Big bloke	Cocaine
Big C	Cocaine
Big D	LSD
Big flake	Cocaine
Big H	Heroin
Big Harry	Heroin
Big O	Opium
Big rush	Cocaine
Bill Blass	Crack
Billie hoke	Cocaine
Bindle	Small packet of drug powder; heroin
Bingers	Crack addicts
Bings	Crack
Birdie powder	Heroin; cocaine
Biscuit	50 rocks of crack
Black	Opium; marijuana
Black acid	LSD; LSD and PCP
Black and white	Amphetamine
Black bart	Marijuana
Black beauties	Depressant; amphetamine
Black birds	Amphetamine
Black bombers	Amphetamine
Black ganga	Marijuana resin
Black gold	High-potency marijuana
Black gungi	Marijuana from India
Black gunion	Marijuana
Black hash	Opium and hashish
Black mo/black moat	Highly potent marijuana
Black mollies	Amphetamine
Black mote	Marijuana mixed with honey
Black pearl	Heroin
Black pill	Opium pill
Black rock	Crack
Black Russian	Hashish mixed with opium
Black star	LSD
Black stuff	Heroin
Black sunshine	LSD
Black tabs	LSD
Black tar	Heroin

Black whack	PCP
Blacks	Amphetamine
Blanco	Heroin
Blanket	Marijuana cigarette
Block	Marijuana
Block busters	Depressant
Blonde	Marijuana
Blotter	LSD; cocaine
Blotter acid	LSD
Blotter cube	LSD
Blow	Cocaine; to inhale cocaine; to smoke marijuana
Blow up	Crack cut with lidocaine to increase size, weight, and street value
Blowcaine	Crack diluted with cocaine
Blowout	Crack
Blud madman	PCP
Blue	Depressant; crack
Blue acid	LSD
Blue angels	Depressant
Blue barrels	LSD
Blue birds	Depressant
Blue boy	Amphetamine
Blue bullets	Depressant
Blue caps	Mescaline
Blue chairs	LSD
Blue cheers	LSD
Blue de hue	Marijuana from Vietnam
Blue devil	Depressant
Blue dolls	Depressant
Blue heaven	LSD
Blue heavens	Depressant
Blue microdot	LSD
Blue mist	LSD
Blue moons	LSD
Blue mystic	2C-T-7
Blue sage	Marijuana
Blue sky blond	High-potency marijuana from Colombia
Blue tips	Depressant
Blue vials	LSD
Blunt	Marijuana inside a cigar; marijuana and cocaine inside a cigar
Bo Bo	Marijuana
Boat	PCP
Bobo	Crack
Bobo bush	Marijuana

Continued

| Table 3 STREET NAMES FOR DRUGS OF ABUSE—CONT'D | |
Street Names	Abused Drug/Interpretation
Bogart a joint	To salivate on a marijuana cigarette; to refuse to share
Bohd	Marijuana; PCP
Bolivian marching powder	Cocaine
Bolo	Crack
Bolt	Isobutyl nitrite
Bomb	Crack; heroin; large marijuana cigarette; high-potency heroin
Bomb squad	Crack-selling crew
Bomber	Marijuana cigarette
Bombido	Injectable amphetamine; heroin; depressant
Bombita	Amphetamine; heroin; depressant
Bombs away	Heroin
Bone	Marijuana; $50 piece of crack
Bonecrusher	Crack
Bones	Crack
Bong	Pipe used to smoke marijuana
Bonita	Heroin
Boo	Marijuana
Boom	Marijuana
Boomers	Psilocybin/psilocin
Boppers	Amyl nitrite
Botray	Crack
Bottles	Crack vials; amphetamine
Boubou	Crack
Boulder	Crack; $20 worth of crack
Boulya	Crack
Bouncing powder	Cocaine
Boy	Heroin
Bozo	Heroin
Brain ticklers	Amphetamine
Brick	1 kilogram of marijuana; crack
Brick gum	Heroin
Britton	Peyote
Broccoli	Marijuana
Brown	Heroin; marijuana
Brown bombers	LSD
Brown crystal	Heroin
Brown dots	LSD
Brown rhine	Heroin
Brown sugar	Heroin
Brownies	Amphetamine
Browns	Amphetamine
Bubble gum	Cocaine; crack

Bud	Marijuana
Buda	A high-grade marijuana joint filled with crack
Bullet	Isobutyl nitrite
Bullia capital	Crack
Bullion	Crack
Bullyon	Marijuana
Bumblebees	Amphetamine
Bump	Crack; fake crack; boost a high; hit of ketamine ($20)
Bundle	Heroin
Bunk	Fake cocaine
Burese	Cocaine
Burnese	Cocaine
Burnie	Marijuana
Bush	Cocaine; marijuana
Businessman's LSD	Dimethyltryptamine
Businessman's special	Dimethyltryptamine
Businessman's trip	Dimethyltryptamine
Busters	Depressant
Busy bee	PCP
Butt naked	PCP
Butter	Marijuana; crack
Butter flower	Marijuana
Buttons	Mescaline
Butu	Heroin
Buzz bomb	Nitrous oxide
C	Cocaine
C, the	Methcathinone
C & M	Cocaine and morphine
C dust	Cocaine
C game	Cocaine
Caballo	Heroin
Cabello	Cocaine
Caca	Heroin
Cactus	Mescaline
Cactus buttons	Mescaline
Cactus head	Mescaline
Cad/Cadillac	1 ounce
Cadillac	PCP
Cadillac express	Methcathinone
Caine	Cocaine; crack
Cakes	Round discs of crack
California cornflakes	Cocaine
California sunshine	LSD
Cam trip	High-potency marijuana
Cambodian red/Cam red	Marijuana from Cambodia

Continued

Table 3 STREET NAMES FOR DRUGS OF ABUSE—CONT'D

Street Names	Abused Drug/Interpretation
Came	Cocaine
Can	Marijuana; 1 ounce
Canadian black	Marijuana
Canamo	Marijuana
Canappa	Marijuana
Cancelled stick	Marijuana cigarette
Candy	Cocaine; crack; depressant; amphetamine
Candy C	Cocaine
Cannabinol	PCP
Cannabis tea	Marijuana
Cap	Crack; LSD
Capital H	Heroin
Caps	Heroin and psilocybin
Carburetor	Crack stem attachment
Carga	Heroin
Carmabis	Marijuana
Carne	Heroin
Carnie	Cocaine
Carrie	Cocaine
Carrie Nation	Cocaine
Cartucho	Package of marijuana cigarettes
Cartwheels	Amphetamine
Casper the ghost	Crack
Cat	Methcathinone
Cat valium	Ketamine
Catnip	Marijuana cigarette
Caviar	Crack
Cavite all-star	Marijuana
Cecil	Cocaine
Chalk	Methamphetamine; amphetamine
Chandoo/chandu	Opium
Charas	Marijuana from India
Charge	Marijuana
Charley	Heroin
Charlie	Cocaine
Chaser	Compulsive crack user
Cheap basing	Crack
Cheeba	Marijuana
Cheeo	Marijuana
Chemical	Crack
Cherry meth	GHB
Chewies	Crack
Chiba chiba	High-potency marijuana from Colombia

Chicago black	Marijuana, term from Chicago
Chicago green	Marijuana
Chicken powder	Amphetamine
Chicle	Heroin
Chief	LSD; mescaline
Chieva	Heroin
China cat	High-potency heroin
China girl	Fentanyl
China town	Fentanyl
China white	Fentanyl
Chinese molasses	Opium
Chinese red	Heroin
Chinese tobacco	Opium
Chip	Heroin
Chippy	Cocaine
Chira	Marijuana
Chocolate	Opium; amphetamine
Chocolate chips	LSD
Chocolate ecstasy	Crack made brown by adding chocolate milk powder during production
Cholly	Cocaine
Chorals	Depressant
Christina	Amphetamine
Christmas rolls	Depressant
Christmas tree	Marijuana; depressant; amphetamine
Chronic	Marijuana; marijuana mixed with crack
Churus	Marijuana
Cid	LSD
Cigarette paper	Packet of heroin
Cigarrode cristal	PCP
Citrol	High-potency marijuana from Nepal
CJ	PCP
Clarity	MDMA (Ecstasy)
Clicker or clickems	Crack and PCP
Cliffhanger	PCP
Climax	Crack; isobutyl nitrite; heroin
Climb	Marijuana cigarette
Cloud	Crack
Cloud nine	Crack
Copilot	Amphetamine
Coasts to coasts	Amphetamine
Coca	Cocaine
Cochornis	Marijuana
Cocktail	Cigarette laced with cocaine or crack; partially smoked marijuana cigarette inserted in regular cigarette

Continued

Table 3 STREET NAMES FOR DRUGS OF ABUSE—CONT'D	
Street Names	**Abused Drug/Interpretation**
Coco rocks	Dark brown crack made by adding chocolate pudding during production
Coco snow	Benzocaine used as cutting agent for crack
Coconut	Cocaine
Coffee	LSD
Coke	Cocaine; crack
Cola	Cocaine
Coli	Marijuana
Coliflor tostado	Marijuana
Colombian	Marijuana
Colorado cocktail	Marijuana
Columbo	PCP
Columbus black	Marijuana
Comeback	Benzocaine and mannitol used to adulterate cocaine for conversion to crack
Conductor	LSD
Contact lens	LSD
Cookies	Crack
Cooler	Cigarette laced with a drug
Coolie	Cigarette laced with cocaine
Coral	Depressant
Corrinne	Cocaine
Cosa	Marijuana
Cotics	Heroin
Cotton brothers	Cocaine, heroin, and morphine
Courage pills	Heroin; depressant
Cozmos	PCP
Crack	Cocaine
Crack back	Crack and marijuana
Crack cooler	Crack soaked in wine cooler
Cracker jacks	Crack smokers
Crackers	LSD
Crank	Methamphetamine; amphetamine; methcathinone
Crap/crop	Low-quality heroin
Crazy coke	PCP
Crazy Eddie	PCP
Crazy weed	Marijuana
Crib	Crack
Crimmie	Cigarette laced with crack
Crink	Methamphetamine
Cripple	Marijuana cigarette
Cris	Methamphetamine
Crisscross	Amphetamine

Cristina	Methamphetamine
Cristy	Smokeable methamphetamine
Croak	Crack and methamphetamine
Cross tops	Amphetamine
Crossroads	Amphetamine
Crown crap	Heroin
Crumbs	Tiny pieces of crack
Crunch & munch	Crack
Cruz	Opium from Vera Cruz, Mexico
Crying weed	Marijuana
Crypto	Methamphetamine
Crystal	Methamphetamine; PCP; amphetamine; cocaine
Crystal joint	PCP
Crystal meth	Methamphetamine
Crystal T	PCP
Crystal tea	LSD
Cube	1 ounce; LSD
Cubes	Marijuana tablets
Culican	High-potency marijuana from Mexico
Cupcakes	LSD
Cura	Heroin
Cut deck	Heroin mixed with powdered milk
Cycline	PCP
Cyclones	PCP
D	LSD, PCP
Dagga	Marijuana
Dama blanca	Cocaine
Dance fever	Fentanyl
Date rape drug/pill	Flunitrazepam (Rohypnol)
Dawamesk	Marijuana
Dead on arrival	Heroin
Decadence	MDMA
Deeda	LSD
Demolish	Crack
DET	Dimethyltryptamine
Detroit pink	PCP
Deuce	$2 worth of drugs; heroin
Devil, the	Crack
Devil's dandruff	Crack
Devil's dick	Crack pipe
Devil's dust	PCP
Devilsmoke	Crack
Dew	Marijuana
Dexies	Amphetamine
Diambista	Marijuana

Continued

Table 3 STREET NAMES FOR DRUGS OF ABUSE—CONT'D

Street Names	Abused Drug/Interpretation
Diet pills	Amphetamine
Dimba	Marijuana from West Africa
Dime	Crack; $10 worth of crack
Dime's worth	Amount of heroin to cause death
Ding	Marijuana
Dinkie dow	Marijuana
Dip	Crack
Dipper	PCP
Dirt	Heroin
Dirt grass	Inferior-quality marijuana
Dirty basing	Crack
Disco biscuits	Depressant
Ditch	Marijuana
Ditch weed	Inferior-quality Mexican marijuana
Djamba	Marijuana
DMT	Dimethyltryptamine
Do it Jack	PCP
DOA	PCP; crack
Doctor	MDMA
Dog food	Heroin
Dogie	Heroin
Dolls	Depressant
Domes	LSD
Domex	PCP and MDMA
Dominoes	Amphetamine
Don jem	Marijuana
Dona Juana	Marijuana
Dona Juanita	Marijuana
Doobie/dubbe/duby	Marijuana
Doogie/doojee/dugie	Heroin
Dooley	Heroin
Dopium	Opium
Doradilla	Marijuana
Dots	LSD
Double bubble	Cocaine
Double cross	Amphetamine
Double dome	LSD
Double rock	Crack diluted with procaine
Double trouble	Depressant
Double ups	A $20 rock that can be broken into and sold as two $20 rocks
Double yoke	Crack
Dove	$35 piece of crack

Dover's powder/Dover's deck	Opium
Downer	Depressant
Downie	Depressant
Draf weed	Marijuana
Drag weed	Marijuana
Dream	Cocaine
Dream gun	Opium
Dream stick	Opium
Dreamer	Morphine
Dreams	Opium
Dreck	Heroin
Drink	PCP
Drowsy high	Depressant
Dry high	Marijuana
Duct	Cocaine
Duji	Heroin
Dummy dust	PCP
Durog	Marijuana
Duros	Marijuana
Dust	Heroin; cocaine; PCP; marijuana mixed with various chemicals
Dust joint	PCP
Dust of angels	PCP
Dusted parsley	PCP
DXM	Dextromethorphan
Dynamite	Heroin and cocaine
Dyno	Heroin
Earth	Marijuana cigarette
Easing powder	Opium
Eastside player	Crack
Easy lay	GHB
Ecstasy	MDMA
Egg	Crack
Eight ball	$\frac{1}{8}$ ounce of drugs
Eighth	Heroin
El diablito	Marijuana, cocaine, heroin, and PCP
El diablo	Marijuana, cocaine, and heroin
Electric Kool Aid	LSD
Elephant	PCP
Elephant tranquilizer	PCP
Embalming fluid	PCP
Emsel	Morphine
Endo	Marijuana
Energizer	PCP
Ephedrone	Methcathinone

Continued

Table 3 STREET NAMES FOR DRUGS OF ABUSE—CONT'D

Street Names	Abused Drug/Interpretation
Erth	PCP
Esra	Marijuana
Essence	MDMA
Estuffa	Heroin
ET	Alpha ethyltryptamine
Eve	MDEA
Everclear	GHB
Eye opener	Crack; amphetamine
Fake STP	PCP
Famous dimes	Crack
Fantasia	Dimethyltryptamine
Fat bags	Crack
Fatty	Marijuana cigarette
Ferry dust	Heroin
Fi-do-nie	Opium
Fields	LSD
Fifty-one	Crack
Fine stuff	Marijuana
Finger	Marijuana cigarette
Fir	Marijuana
First line	Morphine
Fish scales	Crack
Fives	Amphetamine
Fizzies	Methadone
Flake	Cocaine
Flakes	PCP
Flame-throwers	Cigarette laced with cocaine and heroin
Flash	LSD
Flat blues	LSD
Flat chunks	Crack cut with benzocaine
Flea powder	Low-purity heroin
Florida snow	Cocaine
Flower	Marijuana
Flower tops	Marijuana
Fly Mexican airlines	To smoke marijuana
Foo foo dust	Cocaine
Foo foo stuff	Heroin; cocaine
Foolish powder	Heroin; cocaine
Footballs	Amphetamine
Forget pill	Flunitrazepam (Rohypnol)
45-minute psychosis	Dimethyltryptamine
Forwards	Amphetamine
Fraho/frajo	Marijuana

Freebase	Smoking cocaine; crack
Freeze	Cocaine; to renege on a drug deal
French blue	Amphetamine
French fries	Crack
Fresh	PCP
Friend	Fentanyl
Fries	Crack
Frios	Marijuana laced with PCP
Frisco special	Cocaine, heroin, and LSD
Frisco speedball	Cocaine, heroin, and LSD
Friskie powder	Cocaine
Fry	Crack, marijuana soaked in formaldehyde
Fry daddy	Crack and marijuana; cigarette laced with crack
Fu	Marijuana
Fuel	Marijuana mixed with insecticides; PCP
G	GHB
G rock	1 gram of rock cocaine
G shot	Small dose of drugs used to hold off withdrawal symptoms until full dose can be taken
G.B.	Depressant
Gaffel	Fake cocaine
Gage/gauge	Marijuana
Gagers	Methcathinone
Galloping horse	Heroin
Gamma	GHB
Gamot	Heroin
Gange	Marijuana
Gangster	Marijuana
Gangster pills	Depressant
Ganja	Marijuana from Jamaica
Gank	Fake crack
Garbage rock	Crack
Gash	Marijuana
Gasper	Marijuana cigarette
Gasper stick	Marijuana cigarette
Gato	Heroin
Gauge butt	Marijuana
Gee	Opium
Geek	Crack and marijuana
George smack	Heroin
Georgia Home Boy	GHB
Ghana	Marijuana
GHB	Gamma hydroxybutyrate
Ghost	LSD
Gift of the sun	Cocaine

Continued

Table 3 STREET NAMES FOR DRUGS OF ABUSE—CONT'D

Street Names	Abused Drug/Interpretation
Giggle smoke	Marijuana
Gimmie	Crack and marijuana
Gin	Cocaine
Girl	Cocaine; crack; heroin
Girlfriend	Cocaine
Glacines	Heroin
Glad stuff	Cocaine
Glading	Using inhalant
Glass	Hypodermic needle; amphetamine
Glo	Crack
Go fast	Methcathinone
God's drug	Morphine
God's flesh	Psilocybin/psilocin
God's medicine	Opium
Gold	Marijuana; crack
Gold dust	Cocaine
Gold star	Marijuana
Golden dragon	LSD
Golden girl	Heroin
Golden leaf	Marijuana, very high quality
Golf ball	Crack
Golf balls	Depressant
Golpe	Heroin
Goma	Opium; black tar heroin
Gondola	Opium
Gong	Marijuana; opium
Goob	Methcathinone
Good	PCP
Good and plenty	Heroin
Good butt	Marijuana cigarette
Good giggles	Marijuana
Good H	Heroin
Goodfellas	Fentanyl
Goof butt	Marijuana cigarette
Goofball	Cocaine and heroin; depressant
Goofers	Depressant
Goofy's	LSD
Goon	PCP
Goon dust	PCP
Goric	Opium
Gorilla biscuits	PCP
Gorilla pills	Depressant
Gorilla tab	PCP
Gram	Hashish

Grape parfait	LSD
Grass	Marijuana
Grass brownies	Marijuana
Grata	Marijuana
Gravel	Crack
Gravy	Heroin
Great bear	Fentanyl
Great Hormones at Bedtime	GHB
Great tobacco	Opium
Green	Inferior-quality marijuana; PCP; ketamine
Green double domes	LSD
Green dragons	Depressant
Green frog	Depressant
Green goddess	Marijuana
Green gold	Cocaine
Green leaves	PCP
Green single domes	LSD
Green tea	PCP
Green wedge	LSD
Greeter	Marijuana
Greta	Marijuana
Grey shields	LSD
Griefo	Marijuana
Grievous Bodily Harm	GHB
Griff	Marijuana
Griffa	Marijuana
G-riffic	GHB
Griffo	Marijuana
Grit	Crack
Groceries	Crack
Gum	Opium
Guma	Opium
Gungun	Marijuana
Gyve	Marijuana cigarette
H	Heroin
H & C	Heroin and cocaine
H Caps	Heroin
Hache	Heroin
Hail	Crack
Hairy	Heroin
Half a football field	50 rocks of crack
Half load	15 bags (decks) of heroin
Half moon	Peyote
Half track	Crack
Hamburger helper	Crack

Continued

Table 3 STREET NAMES FOR DRUGS OF ABUSE—CONT'D

Street Names	Abused Drug/Interpretation
Hanhich	Marijuana
Hanyak	Smokeable speed
Happy cigarette	Marijuana cigarette
Happy dust	Cocaine
Happy powder	Cocaine
Happy trails	Cocaine
Hard candy	Heroin
Hard line	Crack
Hard rock	Crack
Hard stuff	Opium; heroin
Hardware	Isobutyl nitrite
Harry	Heroin
Has	Marijuana
Hats	LSD
Have a dust	Cocaine
Haven dust	Cocaine
Hawaiian	Marijuana, very high potency
Hawaiian sunshine	LSD
Hawk	LSD
Hay	Marijuana
Hay butt	Marijuana cigarette
Haze	LSD
Hazel	Heroin
HCP	PCP
He man	Fentanyl
Head drugs	Amphetamine
Headlights	LSD
Hearts	Amphetamine
Heaven and hell	PCP
Heaven dust	Heroin; cocaine
Heavenly blue	LSD
Helen	Heroin
Hell dust	Heroin
Hemp	Marijuana
Henry	Heroin
Henry VIII	Cocaine
Her	Cocaine
Herb	Marijuana
Herb and Al	Marijuana and alcohol
Herba	Marijuana
Herms	PCP
Hero	Heroin
Hero of the underworld	Heroin

Heroina	Heroin
Herone	Heroin
Hessle	Heroin
Hikori	Peyote
Hikuli	Peyote
Him	Heroin
Hinkley	PCP
Hiropon	Smokeable methamphetamine
Hit	Crack; marijuana cigarette; to smoke marijuana
Hocus	Opium; marijuana
Hog	PCP
Hombre	Heroin
Hombrecitos	Psilocybin
Homegrown	Marijuana
Honey blunts	Marijuana cigars sealed with honey
Honey oil	Ketamine; inhalant
Hong yen	Heroin in pill form
Hooch	Marijuana
Hooter	Cocaine; marijuana
Hop/hops	Opium
Horning	Heroin; to inhale cocaine
Horse	Heroin
Horse heads	Amphetamine
Horse tracks	PCP
Horse tranquilizer	PCP
Hot dope	Heroin
Hot ice	Smokeable methamphetamine
Hot load/hot shot	Lethal injection of an opiate
Hot stick	Marijuana cigarette
Hotcakes	Crack
How do you like me now?	Crack
Hows	Morphine
HRN	Heroin
Hubba, I am back	Crack
Hubbas	Crack, term from Northern California
Huffer	Inhalant abuser
Hunter	Cocaine
Hyatari	Peyote
I am back	Crack
Ice	Cocaine; methamphetamine; smokeable amphetamine; MDMA; PCP
Ice cube	Crack
Icing	Cocaine
Idiot pills	Depressant
In-betweens	Depressant; amphetamine

Continued

Table 3 STREET NAMES FOR DRUGS OF ABUSE—CONT'D

Street Names	Abused Drug/Interpretation
Inca message	Cocaine
Indian boy	Marijuana
Indian hay	Marijuana from India
Indo	Marijuana, term from Northern California
Indonesian bud	Marijuana; opium
Instant zen	LSD
Isda	Heroin
Issues	Crack
J	Marijuana cigarette
Jackpot	Fentanyl
Jam	Amphetamine; cocaine
Jam cecil	Amphetamine
Jane	Marijuana
Jay	Marijuana cigarette
Jay smoke	Marijuana
Jee gee	Heroin
Jellies	Depressant
Jelly	Cocaine
Jelly baby	Amphetamine
Jelly bean	Amphetamine; depressant
Jelly beans	Crack
Jet	Ketamine
Jet fuel	PCP
Jim Jones	Marijuana laced with cocaine and PCP
Jive	Heroin; marijuana; drugs
Jive doo jee	Heroin
Jive stick	Marijuana
Johnson	Crack
Joint	Marijuana cigarette
Jojee	Heroin
Jolly bean	Amphetamine
Jolly green	Marijuana
Jones	Heroin
Joy flakes	Heroin
Joy juice	Depressant
Joy plant	Opium
Joy powder	Heroin; cocaine
Joy smoke	Marijuana
Joy stick	Marijuana cigarette
Ju ju	Marijuana cigarette
Juan Valdez	Marijuana
Juanita	Marijuana
Jugs	Amphetamine

Juice	Steroids; PCP
Juice joint	Marijuana cigarette sprinkled with crack
Jum	Sealed plastic bag containing crack
Jumbos	Large vials of crack sold on the streets
Junk	Cocaine; heroin
K	PCP
K blast	PCP
K hole	Periods of ketamine-induced confusion
Kabayo	Heroin
Kaksonjae	Smokeable methamphetamine
Kali	Marijuana
Kangaroo	Crack
Kaps	PCP
Karachi	Heroin
Kaya	Marijuana
Kentucky blue	Marijuana
KGB (killer green bud)	Marijuana
Kibbles & bits	Small crumbs of crack
Kick stick	Marijuana cigarette
Kiddie dope	Prescription drugs
Kiff	Marijuana
Killer	Marijuana; PCP
Killer weed (1960s)	Marijuana
Killer weed (1980s)	Marijuana and PCP
Kilter	Marijuana
Kind	Marijuana
King ivory	Fentanyl
King Kong pills	Depressant
King's habit	Cocaine
Kit Kat	Ketamine
KJ	PCP
Kleenex	MDMA
Klingons	Crack addicts
Kokomo	Crack
Koller joints	PCP
Kona gold	Marijuana from Hawaii
Kools	PCP
Kryptonite	Crack
Krystal	PCP
Krystal joint	PCP
Kumba	Marijuana
KW	PCP
L	LSD
L.A.	Long-acting amphetamine
L.A. glass	Smokeable methamphetamine

Continued

Table 3 STREET NAMES FOR DRUGS OF ABUSE—CONT'D	
Street Names	**Abused Drug/Interpretation**
L.A. ice	Smokeable methamphetamine
L.L.	Marijuana
La rocha	Flunitrazepam (Rohypnol)
Lace	Cocaine and marijuana
Lady	Cocaine
Lady caine	Cocaine
Lady snow	Cocaine
Lakbay diva	Marijuana
Las mujercitas	Psilocybin
Lason sa daga	LSD
Laughing gas	Nitrous oxide
Laughing grass	Marijuana
Laughing weed	Marijuana
Lay back	Depressant
LBJ	LSD; PCP; heroin
Leaf	Marijuana; cocaine
Leaky bolla	PCP
Leaky leak	PCP
Leapers	Amphetamine
Lemon 714	PCP
Lemonade	Heroin; poor-quality drugs
Lens	LSD
Lethal weapon	PCP
Lib (Librium)	Depressant
Lid	1 ounce of marijuana
Lid proppers	Amphetamine
Light stuff	Marijuana
Lightning	Amphetamine
Lima	Marijuana
Lime acid	LSD
Line	Cocaine
Little bomb	Amphetamine; heroin; depressant
Little ones	PCP
Little smoke	Marijuana; psilocybin/psilocin
Live ones	PCP
Llesca	Marijuana
Load	25 bags of heroin
Loaf	Marijuana
Lobo	Marijuana
Locker room	Isobutyl nitrite
Locoweed	Marijuana
Log	PCP; marijuana cigarette
Logor	LSD

Love	Crack
Love affair	Cocaine
Love boat	Marijuana dipped in formaldehyde; PCP
Love drug	MDMA; depressant
Love pearls	Alpha ethyltryptamine
Love pills	Alpha ethyltryptamine
Love trip	MDMA and mescaline
Love weed	Marijuana
Lovelies	Marijuana laced with PCP
Lovely	PCP
LSD	Lysergic acid diethylamide
Lubage	Marijuana
Lucy in the sky with diamonds	LSD
Ludes	Depressant (quaaludes)
Luding out	Depressant
Luds	Depressant
M	Marijuana; morphine
M&M	Depressant
M.J.	Marijuana
M.O.	Marijuana
M.S.	Morphine
M.U.	Marijuana
Machinery	Marijuana
Macon	Marijuana
Mad dog	PCP
Madman	PCP
Magic	PCP
Magic dust	PCP
Magic mushroom	Psilocybin/psilocin
Magic smoke	Marijuana
Malcom X	Ketamine
Mama coca	Cocaine
Manhattan silver	Marijuana
Marathons	Amphetamine
Mari	Marijuana cigarette
Marshmallow reds	Depressant
Mary	Marijuana
Mary and Johnny	Marijuana
Mary Ann	Marijuana
Mary Jane	Marijuana
Mary Jonas	Marijuana
Mary Warner	Marijuana
Mary Weaver	Marijuana
Matchbox	¼ ounce of marijuana or 6 marijuana cigarettes
Matsakow	Heroin

Continued

Table 3 STREET NAMES FOR DRUGS OF ABUSE—CONT'D	
Street Names	**Abused Drug/Interpretation**
Maui wauie	Marijuana from Hawaii
Max	GHB dissolved in water and mixed with amphetamines
Mayo	Cocaine; heroin
MDM	MDMA
MDMA	Methylenedioxy methamphetamine
Mean green	PCP
Meg	Marijuana
Megg	Marijuana cigarette
Meggie	Marijuana
Mellow yellow	LSD
Merk	Cocaine
Mesc	Mescaline
Mescal	Mescaline
Mese	Mescaline
Messorole	Marijuana
Meth	Methamphetamine
Mexican brown	Heroin; marijuana
Mexican horse	Heroin
Mexican mud	Heroin
Mexican mushroom	Psilocybin/psilocin
Mexican red	Marijuana
Mexican reds	Depressant
Mezc	Mescaline
Mickey Finn	Depressant
Mickey's	Depressant
Microdot	LSD
Midnight oil	Opium
Mighty Joe Young	Depressant
Mighty mezz	Marijuana cigarette
Mighty Quinn	LSD
Mind detergent	LSD
Minibennie	Amphetamine
Mint leaf	PCP
Mint weed	PCP
Mira	Opium
Miss Emma	Morphine
Missile basing	Crack liquid and PCP
Mist	PCP; crack smoke
Mister blue	Morphine
Modams	Marijuana
Mohasky	Marijuana
Mojo	Cocaine; heroin

Monkey	Cigarette made from cocaine paste and tobacco
Monkey dust	PCP
Monkey tranquilizer	PCP
Monos	Cigarette made from cocaine paste and tobacco
Monte	Marijuana from South America
Mooca/moocah	Marijuana
Moon	Mescaline
Moonrock	Crack and heroin
Mooster	Marijuana
Moota/mutah	Marijuana
Mooters	Marijuana cigarette
Mootie	Marijuana
Mootos	Marijuana
Mor a grifa	Marijuana
More	PCP
Morf	Morphine
Morotgara	Heroin
Mortal combat	High-potency heroin
Mosquitos	Cocaine
Mota/moto	Marijuana
Mother	Marijuana
Mother's little helper	Depressant
Movie star drug	Cocaine
Mud	Opium; heroin
Muggie	Marijuana
Mujer	Cocaine
Murder 8	Fentanyl
Murder one	Heroin and cocaine
Mushrooms	Psilocybin/psilocin
Musk	Psilocybin/psilocin
Mutha	Marijuana
Muzzle	Heroin
Nail	Marijuana cigarette
Nanoo	Heroin
Nebbies	Depressant
Nemmies	Depressant
New acid	PCP
New Jack Swing	Heroin and morphine
New magic	PCP
Nice and easy	Heroin
Nickel bag	$5 worth of drugs; heroin
Nickel deck	Heroin
Niebla	PCP
Nimbies	Depressant
Noise	Heroin

Continued

Table 3 STREET NAMES FOR DRUGS OF ABUSE—CONT'D

Street Names	Abused Drug/Interpretation
Nose	Heroin
Nose candy	Cocaine
Nose drops	Heroin, liquefied
Nose powder	Cocaine
Nose stuff	Cocaine
Nubs	Peyote
Nugget	Amphetamine
Nuggets	Crack
Number	Marijuana cigarette
Number 3	Cocaine, heroin
Number 4	Heroin
Number 8	Heroin
O	Opium
O.J.	Marijuana
O.P.	Opium
O.P.P.	PCP
Octane	PCP laced with gasoline
Ogoy	Heroin
Oil	Heroin, PCP
Old Steve	Heroin
One box tissue	1 ounce of crack
One fifty one	Crack
One way	LSD
Ope	Opium
Optical illusions	LSD
Orange barrels	LSD
Orange crystal	PCP
Orange cubes	LSD
Orange haze	LSD
Orange micro	LSD
Orange wedges	LSD
Oranges	Amphetamine
Outer limits	Crack and LSD
Owsley	LSD
Owsley's acid	LSD
Ozone	PCP
P	Peyote; PCP
P dope	20% to 30% pure heroin
P Funk	Heroin; crack and PCP
P.R. (Panama Red)	Marijuana
Pack	Heroin; marijuana
Pack of rocks	Marijuana cigarette
Pakalolo	Marijuana

Pakistani black	Marijuana
Panama cut	Marijuana
Panama gold	Marijuana
Panama red	Marijuana
Panatella	Large marijuana cigarette
Pancakes and syrup	Combination of glutethimide and codeine cough syrup
Pane	LSD
Pangonadalot	Heroin
Paper acid	LSD
Paper blunts	Marijuana within a paper casing rather than a tobacco-leaf casing
Parachute	Crack and PCP smoked; heroin
Paradise	Cocaine
Paradise white	Cocaine
Parlay	Crack
Parsley	Marijuana; PCP
Paste	Crack
Pat	Marijuana
Patico	Crack (Spanish)
Paz	PCP
PCP	Phencyclidine
PCPA	PCP
Peace	LSD; PCP
Peace pill	PCP
Peace tablets	LSD
Peace weed	PCP
Peaches	Amphetamine
Peanut	Depressant
Peanut butter	PCP mixed with peanut butter
Pearl	Cocaine
Pearls	Amyl nitrite
Pearly gates	LSD
Pebbles	Crack
Pee Wee	Crack; $5 worth of crack
Peep	PCP
Peg	Heroin
Pellets	LSD
Pen yan	Opium
Pep pills	Amphetamine
Perfect high	Heroin
Perico	Cocaine
Perp	Fake crack made of candle wax and baking soda
Peruvian	Cocaine
Peruvian flake	Cocaine
Peruvian lady	Cocaine

Continued

Table 3 STREET NAMES FOR DRUGS OF ABUSE—CONT'D

Street Names	Abused Drug/Interpretation
Peter Pan	PCP
Peth	Depressant
Peyote	Mescaline
Phennies	Depressant
Phenos	Depressant
Piedras	Crack (Spanish)
Pig killer	PCP
Piles	Crack
Pimp	Cocaine
Pin	Marijuana
Pin gon	Opium
Pin yen	Opium
Pink blotters	LSD
Pink hearts	Amphetamine
Pink ladies	Depressant
Pink Panther	LSD
Pink robots	LSD
Pink wedge	LSD
Pink witches	LSD
Pit	PCP
Pixies	Amphetamine
Pocket rocket	Marijuana
Pod	Marijuana
Poison	Heroin; fentanyl
Poke	Marijuana
Polvo	Heroin; PCP
Polvo blanco	Cocaine
Polvo de angel	PCP
Polvo de estrellas	PCP
Pony	Crack
Poppers	Isobutyl nitrite; amyl nitrite
Poppy	Heroin
Pot	Marijuana
Potato	LSD
Potato chips	Crack cut with benzocaine
Potten bush	Marijuana
Powder	Heroin; amphetamine
Powder diamonds	Cocaine
Pox	Opium
Prescription	Marijuana cigarette
Press	Cocaine; crack
Pretendica	Marijuana
Pretendo	Marijuana

Primo	Crack; marijuana mixed with crack
Primos	Cigarettes laced with cocaine and heroin
Pseudocaine	Phenylpropanolamine, an adulterant for cutting crack
Puffer	Crack smoker
Puffy	PCP
Pulborn	Heroin
Pure	Heroin
Pure love	LSD
Purple	Ketamine
Purple barrels	LSD
Purple flats	LSD
Purple haze	LSD
Purple hearts	LSD; amphetamine; depressant
Purple ozoline	LSD
Purple rain	PCP
Q	Depressant
Quad	Depressant
Quarter moon	Hashish
Quartz	Smokeable speed
Quas	Depressant
Queen Anne's lace	Marijuana
Quicksilver	Isobutyl nitrite
Quill	Methamphetamine; heroin; cocaine
R-2	Flunitrazepam (Rohypnol)
Racehorse charlie	Cocaine; heroin
Ragweed	Inferior quality marijuana; heroin
Railroad weed	Marijuana
Rainbows	Depressant
Rainy day woman	Marijuana
Rambo	Heroin
Rane	Cocaine; heroin
Rangood	Marijuana grown wild
Rasta weed	Marijuana
Raw	Crack
Ready rock	Cocaine; crack; heroin
Recycle	LSD
Red and blue	Depressant
Red bullets	Depressant
Red caps	Crack
Red chicken	Heroin
Red cross	Marijuana
Red devil	Depressant; PCP
Red dirt	Marijuana
Red eagle	Heroin
Red phosphorus	Smokeable speed

Continued

Table 3 STREET NAMES FOR DRUGS OF ABUSE—CONT'D

Street Names	Abused Drug/Interpretation
Reds	Depressant
Reefer	Marijuana
Regular P	Crack
Reindeer dust	Heroin
Rhine	Heroin
Rhythm	Amphetamine
Rib	Flunitrazepam (Rohypnol)
Rib Roche	Flunitrazepam (Rohypnol)
Righteous bush	Marijuana
Rippers	Amphetamine
Roache-2, Roaches, Roachies	Flunitrazepam (Rohypnol)
Road dope	Amphetamine
Roca	Crack (Spanish)
Rocha	Flunitrazepam (Rohypnol)
Roche, Roches	Flunitrazepam (Rohypnol)
Rock attack	Crack
Rock(s)	Cocaine; crack
Rocket fuel	PCP
Rockets	Marijuana cigarette
Rocks of hell	Crack
Rocky III	Crack
Rolling	MDMA
Rooster	Crack
Root	Marijuana
Rope	Marijuana; flunitrazepam (Rohypnol)
Rosa	Amphetamine
Rose Marie	Marijuana
Roses	Amphetamine
Rox	Crack
Roxanne	Cocaine; crack
Royal blues	LSD
Roz	Crack
Running	MDMA
Rush	Isobutyl nitrite
Rush snappers	Isobutyl nitrite
Russian sickles	LSD
Sack	Heroin
Sacrament	LSD
Sacred mushroom	Psilocybin
Salt	Heroin
Salt and pepper	Marijuana
Salty water	GHB
Sandoz	LSD

Sandwich	Two layers of cocaine with a layer of heroin in the middle
Santa Marta	Marijuana
Sasfras	Marijuana
Scaffle	PCP
Scag	Heroin
Scat	Heroin
Scate	Heroin
Schmeck	Cocaine
Schoolboy	Cocaine, codeine
Schoolcraft	Crack
Scissors	Marijuana
Score	Purchase drugs
Scorpion	Cocaine
Scott	Heroin
Scottie	Cocaine
Scotty	Cocaine; crack; the high from crack
Scramble	Crack
Scruples	Crack
Scuffle	PCP
Seccy	Depressant
Seeds	Marijuana
Seggy	Depressant
Sen	Marijuana
Seni	Peyote
Sernyl	PCP
Serpico 21	Cocaine
Sess	Marijuana
Seven-up	Cocaine; crack
Sezz	Marijuana
Shake	Marijuana
She	Cocaine
Sheet rocking	Crack and LSD
Sheets	PCP
Shermans	PCP
Sherms	PCP; crack; marijuana soaked in formaldehyde
Shmeck/schmeek	Heroin
Shoot the breeze	Nitrous oxide
Shrooms	Psilocybin/psilocin
Siddi	Marijuana
Sightball	Crack
Silly Putty	Psilocybin/psilocin
Simple Simon	Psilocybin/psilocin
Sinse	Marijuana
Sinsemilla	Potent variety of marijuana

Continued

Table 3 STREET NAMES FOR DRUGS OF ABUSE—CONT'D	
Street Names	**Abused Drug/Interpretation**
Sixty-two	2½ ounces of crack
Skee	Opium
Skid	Heroin
Skuffle	PCP
Skunk	Marijuana
Slab	Crack
Sleeper	Heroin; depressant
Sleet	Crack
Slick superspeed	Methcathinone
Slime	Heroin
Smack	Heroin
Smears	LSD
Smoke	Heroin and crack; crack; marijuana
Smoke Canada	Marijuana
Smoking	PCP
Smoking gun	Heroin and cocaine
Snap	Amphetamine
Snappers	Isobutyl nitrite
Snop	Marijuana
Snorts	PCP
Snow	Cocaine; heroin; amphetamine
Snow bird	Cocaine
Snow pallets	Amphetamine
Snow seals	Cocaine and amphetamine
Snow soke	Crack
Snow white	Cocaine
Snowball	Cocaine and heroin
Snowcones	Cocaine
Society high	Cocaine
Soda	Injectable cocaine used in Latino communities
Softballs	Depressant
Soles	Hashish
Soma	PCP
Sopers	Depressant
Space base	Crack dipped in PCP; hollowed-out cigar refilled with PCP and crack
Space cadet	Crack dipped in PCP
Space dust	Crack dipped in PCP
Sparkle plenty	Amphetamine
Sparklers	Amphetamine
Special "K"	Ketamine
Special la coke	Ketamine
Speed	Methamphetamine; amphetamine; crack

Speed boat	Marijuana, PCP, crack
Speed for lovers	MDMA
Speedball	Heroin and cocaine (IV); amphetamine
Spider blue	Heroin
Splash	Amphetamine
Spliff	Marijuana cigarette
Splim	Marijuana
Splivins	Amphetamine
Spores	PCP
Square mackerel	Marijuana, term from Florida
Square time Bob	Crack
Squirrel	Smoking cocaine, marijuana and PCP; LSD
Stack	Marijuana
Star	Methcathinone
Star-spangled powder	Cocaine
Stardust	Cocaine, PCP
Stat	Methcathinone
Stems	Marijuana
Stick	Marijuana, PCP
Stink weed	Marijuana
Stones	Crack
Stoppers	Depressant
STP	PCP
Straw	Marijuana cigarette
Strawberry fields	LSD
Stuff	Heroin
Stumbler	Depressant
Sugar	Cocaine; LSD; heroin
Sugar block	Crack
Sugar cubes	LSD
Sugar lumps	LSD
Sugar weed	Marijuana
Sunshine	LSD
Super	PCP
Super acid	Ketamine
Super C	Ketamine
Super grass	PCP
Super ice	Smokeable methamphetamine
Super joint	PCP
Super kools	PCP
Super weed	PCP
Supergrass	Marijuana
Surfer	PCP
Sweet Jesus	Heroin
Sweet Lucy	Marijuana

Continued

Table 3 STREET NAMES FOR DRUGS OF ABUSE—CONT'D

Street Names	Abused Drug/Interpretation
Sweet stuff	Heroin; cocaine
Sweets	Amphetamine
Swell up	Crack
Synthetic cocaine	PCP
Synthetic THT	PCP
T	Cocaine; marijuana
T7	2C-T-7
T buzz	PCP
T.N.T.	Heroin; fentanyl
Tabs	LSD
Tail lights	LSD
Taima	Marijuana
Taking a cruise	PCP
Takkouri	Marijuana
Tango & Cash	Fentanyl
Tar	Opium; heroin
Tardust	Cocaine
Taste	Heroin; small sample of drugs
Tea	Marijuana, PCP
Tecate	Heroin
Teener	$\frac{1}{16}$ ounce of methamphetamine
Teeth	Cocaine; crack
Tension	Crack
Tex mex	Marijuana
Texas pot	Marijuana
Texas shoe shine	Spray paint containing toluene
Texas tea	Marijuana
Thai sticks	Bundles of marijuana soaked in hashish oil; marijuana buds bound on short sections of bamboo
THC	Tetrahydrocannabinol
Thirteen	Marijuana
Thrust	Isobutyl nitrite
Thrusters	Amphetamine
Thumb	Marijuana
Tic	PCP in powder form
Tic tac	PCP
Ticket	LSD
Tish	PCP
Tissue	Crack
Titch	PCP
Toncho	Octane booster that is inhaled
Tooles	Depressant
Toot	Cocaine; to inhale cocaine

Tooties	Depressant
Tootsie roll	Heroin
Top gun	Crack
Topi	Mescaline
Tops	Peyote
Torch	Marijuana
Torch up	To smoke marijuana
Torpedo	Crack and marijuana
Totally spent	MDMA hangover
Toxy	Opium
Toys	Opium
TR 6s	Amphetamine
Tragic magic	Crack dipped in PCP
Trank	PCP
Tranq	Depressant
Trip	LSD; alpha ethyltryptamine
Troop	Crack
Truck drivers	Amphetamine
TT1	PCP
TT2	PCP
TT3	PCP
Tuie	Depressant
Turbo	Crack and marijuana
Turkey	Cocaine; amphetamine
Turnabout	Amphetamine
Tutti frutti	Flavored cocaine developed by a Brazilian gang
Tweek	Methamphetamine-like substance
Tweeker	Methcathinone
Twenty-five	LSD
Twist	Marijuana cigarette
Twistum	Marijuana cigarette
Ultimate	Crack
Uncle Milty	Depressant
Unkie	Morphine
Uppers	Amphetamine
Uppies	Amphetamine
Ups and downs	Depressant
Utopiates	Hallucinogens
Uzi	Crack; crack pipe
V	Valium
Viper's weed	Marijuana
Vitamin K	Ketamine
Vodka acid	LSD
Wac	PCP on marijuana
Wack	PCP

Continued

Table 3 STREET NAMES FOR DRUGS OF ABUSE—CONT'D

Street Names	Abused Drug/Interpretation
Wacky weed	Marijuana
Wake ups	Amphetamine
Water	Methamphetamine, PCP
Wave	Crack
Wedding bells	LSD
Wedge	LSD
Weed	Marijuana, PCP
Weed tea	Marijuana
Whack	PCP and heroin
Wheat	Marijuana
When shee	Opium
Whippets	Nitrous oxide
White	Amphetamine
White ball	Crack
White boy	Heroin
White cross	Methamphetamine; amphetamine
White dust	LSD
White ghost	Crack
White girl	Cocaine; heroin
White-haired lady	Marijuana
White horizon	PCP
White horse	Cocaine
White junk	Heroin
White lady	Cocaine; heroin
White lightning	LSD
White mosquito	Cocaine
White nurse	Heroin
White Owsley's	LSD
White powder	Cocaine; PCP
White stuff	Heroin
White sugar	Crack
White tornado	Crack
Whiteout	Isobutyl nitrite
Whites	Amphetamine
Whiz bang	Cocaine and heroin
Wild cat	Methcathinone and cocaine
Window glass	LSD
Window pane	LSD
Wings	Heroin; cocaine
Witch	Heroin; cocaine
Witch hazel	Heroin
Wobble weed	PCP
Wolf	PCP

Wollie	Rocks of crack rolled into a marijuana cigarette
Woolah	A hollowed-out cigar refilled with marijuana and crack
Woolas	Cigarette laced with cocaine; marijuana cigarette sprinkled with crack
Woolies	Marijuana and crack or PCP
Wooly blunts	Marijuana and crack or PCP
Worm	PCP
Wrecking crew	Crack
X	Marijuana; MDMA; amphetamine
X ing	MDMA
XTC	MDMA
Yahoo/yeaho	Crack
Yale	Crack
Yeh	Marijuana
Yellow	LSD; depressant
Yellow bam	Methamphetamine
Yellow bullets	Depressant
Yellow dimples	LSD
Yellow fever	PCP
Yellow jackets	Depressant
Yellow submarine	Marijuana
Yellow sunshine	LSD
Yen pop	Marijuana
Yen Shee Suey	Opium wine
Yerba	Marijuana
Yerba mala	PCP and marijuana
Yesca	Marijuana
Yesco	Marijuana
Yeyo	Cocaine, Spanish term
Yimyom	Crack
Z	1 ounce of heroin
Zacatecas purple	Marijuana from Mexico
Zambi	Marijuana
Ze	Opium
Zen	LSD
Zero	Opium
Zig zag man	LSD; marijuana; marijuana rolling papers
Zip	Cocaine; smokeable methamphetamine
Zol	Marijuana cigarette
Zombie	PCP; heavy user of drugs
Zombie weed	PCP
Zoom	PCP; marijuana laced with PCP

Appendix E

Adverse Effect Monitoring

Carson R. Harris

Table 4 provides a list of adverse effects found with common drugs of abuse that you should be aware of, especially in the admitted patient.

Table 4 ADVERSE EFFECTS OF COMMON DRUGS OF ABUSE

Drug	Adverse Effects to Monitor
Amyl nitrite	Headache, flushing, nausea, vomiting, hypotension, methemoglobinemia
Amphetamines	Anxiety, agitation, seizures, hypertension, tachycardia, intracranial hemorrhage, vasospasm, hyperthermia, rhabdomyolysis
Cocaine	Agitation, hyperexcitability, hypertension, seizures, tachycardia, v. tach, v. fib, coronary artery spasm, thrombosis, rhabdomyolysis, hyperthermia
Fentanyl	Pinpoint pupils, respiratory depression, CNS depression
GHB	Sedation, respiratory depression (especially in large doses or when mixed with other depressants like alcohol), coma, seizures
Heroin	Pinpoint pupils, respiratory depression, CNS depression, pulmonary edema
Isobutyl nitrite	Headache, flushing, nausea, vomiting, hypotension, methemoglobinemia, v. fib
Ketamine	Dyskinesias, hallucinations, delirium, hypertension or hypotension, seizures, cardiac arrhythmias, respiratory stimulation or depression
Klonopin	Respiratory depression, CNS depression, lethargy, slurred speech, ataxia, coma
LSD	Anxiety, psychosis, paranoia, seizures, severe hyperthermia, hypertension, cardiac arrhythmias, rhabdomyolysis

Marijuana	Euphoria, altered time perception, visual hallucinations and agitation (have been seen more recently); hypotension and tachycardia possible
MDMA	Agitation, bruxism, hypertension, tachycardia, hyperthermia, seizures
Methamphetamines	Anxiety, agitation, seizures, hypertension, tachycardia, cardiac arrhythmias, hyperthermia, rhabdomyolysis, seizures
Morphine	Pinpoint pupils, CNS depression, respiratory depression, pulmonary edema
Opium	Pinpoint pupils, CNS depression, respiratory depression, pulmonary edema
PCP	Loss of pain perception, euphoria, hallucinations, bizarre behavior, vertical and horizontal nystagmus, alternating clinical presentation between quiet catatonia and agitated, loud behavior
Psilocybin	Agitation, hallucinations

Index